Fibromyalgia Chronic Fatigue & Irritable Bowel

Treating Symptoms
Treating Cause

Second Edition

Gregory K. Penniston, D.C.

Nonplus Press
Tucson, Arizona

ISBN   0-9785453-0-3

Library of Congress Number: 2006904072

Nonplus Press
6563 E. 22nd St.
Tucson, AZ 85710
Toll Free: (877) 203-4495

Printed in the United States Of America

To the millions of people with nonplus conditions

who have been searching years or even decades

for answers, I hope you find them here.

Contents

Quick Treatment Reference

It is common for fibromyalgia, chronic fatigue and irritable bowel to occur together, although the symptoms of only one of these is likely to be dominant. In addition to these three conditions, there are at least seven other lesser-known conditions that are related to and often occur along with fibromyalgia, chronic fatigue, and irritable bowel. These conditions are Ehlers-Danlos Syndrome, chronic fatigue with immune dysfunction, interstitial cystitis, multiple chemical sensitivity, neurally mediated hypotension, restless legs syndrome and vulvodynia. Each of these conditions are described in chapter 11, Defining the Nonplus Conditions. Unless the symptoms of these conditions are severe, and create a significant disruption of normal life, people are apt to believe that the symptoms they are experiencing, although not normal for most people, are a quirk of their own body that they just have to get used to. Because of this, the symptoms caused by these conditions may be lived with year after year with little complaint or discussion.

Because these conditions share many traits including a favorable response to guaifenesin therapy, I use one name, the nonplus conditions, to refer to this group of related conditions. Guaifenesin is an inexpensive and safe nonprescription medication commonly used as an expectorant. Guaifenesin appears to treat the cause of the nonplus conditions because, in many individuals, it gradually decreases or eliminates all symptoms that result from them.

If you have been diagnosed with one or more of the nonplus conditions, here are the four basic steps to using guaifenesin in a nutshell. Please consult with a physician before using this or any other treatment.

1. **Recognizing all of the symptoms resulting from the nonplus conditions.** In most instances people are not aware of the wide-ranging

symptoms that can be caused by the nonplus conditions. The Symptom Summary Sheet lists over 50 of the most common symptoms. Filling out the Symptom Summary Sheet helps people to recognize, often for the first time, how many of the symptoms they commonly experience are interrelated. Awareness of the symptoms that are caused by the nonplus conditions is important, because once guaifenesin is started, it is changes in the intensity or frequency of these symptoms that indicate when the correct dose has been reached. Guaifenesin may also cause the temporary return of symptoms that have not been experienced in many years. This is another indicator that guaifenesin is reversing the underlying cause of fibromyalgia.

The majority of the symptoms on The Symptom Summary Sheet can have more than one cause. This makes it possible for some of the symptoms on this sheet to be due to health problems other than the nonplus conditions. However, if you can answer yes to the following three statements, then it is likely that the symptom you have marked is due to a nonplus condition.

- Your doctor has ruled out other health problems as the cause of this symptom.
- There is no obvious reason for this symptom.
- Treating this symptom has resulted in little long-term benefit.

The Symptom Summary Sheet makes it much easier to keep track of the changes in the dozens of possible symptoms associated with the nonplus conditions. When filling it out, please take your time, considering each symptom, and then labeling it per the instructions. When people race through filling out this form, they often mislabel symptoms that seem unimportant. By concentrating for a moment on each symptom, will you be more apt to correctly label a symptom. This is especially true for the symptoms that you used to have, but have not experienced for some time. When guaifenesin is started, these previously forgotten symptoms may help you to recognize when the correct dose of guaifenesin has been reached.

2. **Salicylates.** Avoiding salicylates both internally and externally

is critical to insure guaifenesin works properly. Salicylates are a type of chemical present in plant extracts and they are also manufactured synthetically for products such as aspirin and sunscreen. Salicylates block guaifenesin's effectiveness when treating the nonplus conditions. Avoiding salicylates involves learning what products need to be replaced with similar products that contain no natural or synthetic salicylates. For some people, this step of eliminating salicylates can result in some symptom improvement even before guaifenesin is started. If a decrease in symptoms does occur when eliminating salicylates, a person should be aware that this indicates that they are especially susceptible. These people should be particularly careful to identify and eliminate all salicylate sources. Extreme salicylate sensitivity is an important finding and is likely to go unrecognized if guaifenesin is used before all salicylate use has stopped. Taking guaifenesin before eliminating salicylates is also likely to cause errors in dosing guaifenesin even for people who are much less sensitive to salicylates.

This step of eliminating salicylate containing products may take just a day or two or several weeks depending upon the individual. The amount of time it takes to complete this step is not particularly important. What is important is that this step be done properly. Chapter 7 goes into much greater detail on this topic.

For lists of salicylate-free products go to the Guai-Support website at www.psha-inc.com/guai-support and click on the Sal-free™ Centre.

3. **Reactive hypoglycemia.** Know how to recognize the symptoms of reactive hypoglycemia, and if necessary restrict sugary and starchy carbohydrates. If you have reactive hypoglycemia, it is not absolutely necessary to be on a low-carbohydrate diet before starting guaifenesin. See Chapter 9.

4. **Dosing guaifenesin.** Once you have filled out the Symptom Summary Sheet and are salicylate free, you may now dose guaifenesin gradually. Start at 200 to 300 milligrams twice a day depending upon the milligram amount of the pill you are using. If you are anxious about the symptom changes that occur once the therapeutic dose if found, you could start even lower. *The ideal dose is found when a significant*

but tolerable change in one or more of your symptoms becomes apparent.
This change for better and or worse will alter the intensity and or the
frequency of these symptoms.

Increase your daily dose by 200 to 300 milligrams each week until
symptom changes occur. Symptom changes usually include a decrease
as well as a temporary increase in symptoms. It is the change in
symptoms that signal guaifenesin is working. If symptoms increase
excessively, you may have exceeded your optimum dose. If this occurs,
decrease your dose until significant but tolerable changes occur that
include improvement of some symptoms. It is not unusual to experience
a dramatic improvement of several symptoms with no symptom
becoming worse for a period of weeks or months. If this happens to
you consider yourself lucky. See Chapter 8 for details on dosing.

Symptom Summary Sheet

Name:_____

Date:_____

Please assign one of the letters below to each symptom:

D: Daily
W: Weekly
M: Monthly
O: Occasionally
U: Used to have
N: Never

_____ Fatigue
_____ Stiffness
_____ Dizziness/Off Balance
_____ Faintness When Seated Or
       Standing
_____ Unrefreshing Sleep
_____ Impaired Concentration
_____ Sweating
_____ Heart Palpitations
_____ Mitral Valve Prolapse
_____ Chest Pain
_____ Pain In/Around Shoulder
       Blade
_____ Frequent Colds, Flu
_____ Sensitive To Touch With
       Pressure
_____ Irritated Eyes
_____ Abnormal Tastes
       (Metallic, Etc.)
_____ Numbness/Tingling/Burning
_____ Leg Cramps
_____ Bloating
_____ Diarrhea
_____ Gas
_____ Constipation
_____ Irritable Bowel Syndrome
_____ Headaches
_____ Growing Pains
_____ Muscle Or Joint Pain
_____ Jaw Joint Pain
_____ Anxiety

_____ Multiple Chemical
       Sensitivities (Fragrances,
       Fresh Newspaper, New
       Paint, Etc.)
_____ Foot Pain/Fallen Arches
_____ Vulvodynia (Vagina Pain)
_____ Pelvic Pain
_____ Pungent Urine
_____ Painful, Frequent Urination
_____ Hunger Tremors
_____ Sugar Cravings
_____ Panic Attacks
_____ Irritability
_____ Nervousness
_____ Depression
_____ Vision Blurring
_____ Cold Hands/Feet
_____ Nasal Congestion
_____ Ringing In Ears
_____ Restless Legs
_____ Weight Changes
_____ Brittle Nails
_____ Loose Joints/Can't Hold
       Adjustment
_____ Hives
_____ Rashes
_____ Itching
_____ Creepy Crawly Skin
_____ Allergies

Introduction

My Perspective As A Patient

Some time around 1987, I finally decided to make a list of all of my own quirky health problems. For years it had seemed that there were always several health issues plaguing me. During this time of my life, new symptoms were developing, and the intermittent health problems I experienced as a teenager and young adult were coming back to an unusual extent. The funny thing was, in many ways I felt I was a healthy person. I had been an athlete in high school and college, and I had continued to be physically active. My weight was average, I did not take medication and for many years I had little reason to see a doctor. I could go for days or weeks feeling great. On the other hand, I was beginning to experience a lot of unexplainable aches, pains and illnesses that would come and go with no regularity, but seemed to be getting worse. Exercise no longer energized me; instead, it was causing exhaustion that could last for days and was increasingly leading to colds and flu.

When I went to doctors, nothing wrong could be found that could explain my symptoms. As time went on, I felt increasingly unnerved by health problems that eluded all attempts of diagnosis and continued in spite of every healthy lifestyle change I made. Even though I was a doctor, I was running out of ideas of what could be wrong, and I no longer knew what to do. It was like my body had a dark side-a physical dark side. Not in an evil sense, but dark because the problems themselves were not obvious to others and could not even be detected by medical tests. In addition, some symptoms were often difficult to explain and others too fleeting and numerous to remember, so for the most part I did not talk about them.

I had a number of symptoms that were becoming more constant and intense enough to really grab my attention. These included sleep difficulties, often with an inability to lie still similar to restless legs, fatigue, a deep ache/numbness under my right shoulder blade or between my shoulders and chemical sensitivities. I had a second group of symptoms that I would experience two to three times a month: colds and bouts with the flu associated with physical exertion, throat clearing that I could not stop even when there was nothing to clear and a terrible itchiness in my arms that occurred without a rash and could keep me up at night. A third group of symptoms were even more intermittent. These symptoms could be intense for several days and then disappear for months. This group of symptoms included blurred vision, chest and throat pressure, dizziness, neck spasms, digestive problems and several others.

In addition to the symptoms themselves, there was another aspect to what I was experiencing that left me feeling especially disoriented. This occurred when a symptom was present just barely above the conscious level. I could go for hours feeling slightly 'off' or irritable before I fully recognized the symptom that was bothering me. It was only after I became consciously aware of the symptom that I would realize it had been there for a while. Sometimes it would feel like the problem had been present for hours and other times for days, but I couldn't be sure.

I know it is common for people to have this type of experience with a slight headache, but for me the symptom could be a feverish feeling of my skin, dizziness, pressure in my throat or chest and pain between my shoulders. I could experience dizziness so mild that I would spend half of the day taking extra steps to catch my balance or find myself bumping into walls for no reason before I would realize that I was feeling a slight dizziness. How does one explain something like this to other people?

There were actually a variety of reasons why I did not discuss my symptoms. Doesn't everyone have some health issues? Furthermore, there were weeks when I felt just fine, and the pain and other symptoms were just barely noticeable or even completely gone. At this point in my life, I was still entering and sometimes winning mountain bike races in my state. I had a successful practice, and I was an involved father and husband. How could anything really be wrong? I did everything I knew to promote physical and mental health, from a whole food diet to giving myself time to relax and rest.

Health care, health maintenance and prevention was much more than a passing interest of mine, it is also my profession. I must admit that as a doctor actively promoting a healthy lifestyle, I found it embarrassing to have so many different problems and no good reason or explanation for having them.

So, it was in 1987 that I decided I would make a list of every symptom that I experienced over the next month. I believed that if I kept track of how I felt and paid attention to the timing of the problems and under what circumstances they occurred, a logical explanation would become obvious. Or, perhaps I could show the list to another doctor who could help me sort things out objectively. Over the next several weeks I did my best to write down all of the different symptoms as they occurred as well as the time of day, what I had been doing and eating.

I actually remember the day, sitting in my office at work, when I saw the papers my list was written on and decided that it was time to analyze my situation. There was neither rhyme nor reason to my list of about 20 different symptoms. The time of day or week and the type of symptoms experienced were random with the exception that extreme fatigue and flu-type symptoms frequently followed physical exertion. When I saw how diverse and how many problems there actually were, I was stunned. I could see that I spent a lot of time ignoring how I really felt. I also recognized for the first time that I was no different from my patients with fibromyalgia, chronic fatigue and chemical sensitivities. The only difference was in the severity and frequency of my symptoms, which was considerably less than for many of my patients with these conditions. I also immediately understood that I was not going to be able to find solutions any easier than my patients who, after all, were using me to help them find solutions. I had treated hundreds of patients by that time who had gone from doctor to doctor year after year looking for long-term solutions that were never found.

My list had helped me to see the truth of what was wrong, but instead of leading to a solution it seemed there was no way out. I realized that I was one of "those" people, people who doctors see, who I was seeing that never seemed to improve that much. People who, just when you think one of their problems are resolved, it returns, or a new symptom inexplicably comes to take its place. I felt I was in medical no man's land with no one who understood my conditions, no promising treatments and little hope. It appeared that this dark side of me was going to remain in the shadows. If I could not fix these problems, I could at least ignore them. I crumpled up my lists of my symptoms and threw them away.

As time went on, I realized that I was not good at ignoring these problems. I was always willing to try a different way to exercise, a new supplement or diet. After all, if I found something that did help me, it might also prove to be helpful for my patients. In the long run, my willingness to try a variety of different therapies taught me a great deal and eventually, 13 years after writing my list, lead me to guaifenesin, a safe readily available nonprescription expectorant. After five years of taking it, I had gradually improved to the point where I was 90 percent recovered.

I know that every person with a nonplus condition experiences symptoms in their own unique way, which may be considerably different from my experience. For the most part, I experienced a gradual increase of most of my symptoms, but sudden onset may occur following an accident, surgery, and emotional upheaval or even after a cold. A nonplus condition may cause just one symptom that is constant or intermittent or create dozens of symptoms in which some are constant and others are intermittent. Do not think that just because your experience and symptoms are somewhat different from mine that you cannot have a nonplus condition.

My Perspective as a Physician

After I had been in practice for several years, I had people coming to see me specifically for fibromyalgia, chronic fatigue and multiple chemical sensitivities. These patients considered me to be an expert or at least very knowledgeable in these conditions. This elevated status that I had attained in their eyes was because I was familiar enough with these conditions to acknowledge their existence and I was willing to try a variety of approaches to help my patients feel better. It is a sad state of affairs when these qualifications are enough for a doctor to be considered expert.

I actually knew very little about these conditions, and I could not find anyone else who did. Information was hard to come by and research articles often only confirmed what doctors in the field already knew, such as the fact that people suffering with these conditions may not get restful sleep. When medical research papers discussed possible causes and treatments, it was consistently contradictory.

The books on these conditions were no more helpful. The majority of them suggesting lifestyle changes that I was already aware of and was using when appropriate.

In the mid 1990s, a doctor I greatly respect referred a patient to me. The patient had moved to the city where I lived and needed follow up care. She had fibromyalgia, chronic fatigue, neurally mediated hypotension (causing her to sometimes feel faint when she stood or sat upright), irritable bowel, chemical sensitivities, and many other associated symptoms. These were problems I often saw in my patients, but had difficulty resolving so I was particularly interested in finding out how the referring doctor was managing her conditions.

I remember being surprised by the treatment regime that he had this patient following, which included almost a dozen different nutritional supplements, several of which were at high, mega vitamin doses. Even though this approach was a common one found in many books and articles on fibromyalgia and chronic fatigue, I was surprised that the referring doctor was taking this nonspecific shot gun type of approach. I had never found that recommending almost every beneficial supplement for a patient to be more effective than carefully selecting specific products for particular symptoms, and-with trial and error-finding what really helps a patient and what does not. Overall, however, the patient was pleased with her treatment, stating that she had improved, even though she was still disabled to the point of being unable to work.

I decided to call this doctor to ask him about fibromyalgia and chronic fatigue to get a better understanding of what these conditions actually were and how best to treat them. After a pause he said, "If you want to know about fibromyalgia, you should get a book on it." I was taken aback by such a curt answer coming from a colleague. I later took this to mean that he did not feel like he had a better handle on these conditions than the rest of us. The problem was that I had already taken his advice by reading books and many conflicting research articles on these conditions. I had also attended seminars that discussed these conditions. About the only thing that everyone agreed on was that these conditions were challenging in almost every respect.

Never could I have imagined that within five years I would find a treatment that was not only effective on most patients, but also treated several other poorly understood and related conditions. Due to my personal health recovery and success with hundreds of my patients using guaifenesin, I am doing everything I can to disseminate information about the nonplus conditions and treatment using guaifenesin. This includes writing this book, treating and educating my patients, lecturing, managing a website, and running a company that formulates and distributes guaifenesin. Because of these efforts, I am in ongoing contact with guaifenesin users worldwide.

Informal discussions about fibromyalgia and chronic fatigue are common between physicians. I think this is because these conditions are a frequent source of frustration. Behind closed doors doctors may vent these frustrations in a surprisingly frank way, and their opinions are not always supportive regarding the patients who have these conditions. I find negative opinions about these conditions and the people who have them may be present even among the most conscientious and qualified doctors. These doctors put a considerable amount of effort into doing their best for patients and are used to having their efforts rewarded by seeing patients improve. Unfortunately, even their best efforts meet with little success when treating fibromyalgia, chronic fatigue, irritable bowel and the other nonplus conditions. The number and variability of the symptoms together with resistance to treatment create an almost irresistible urge to believe that these patients have emotional or psychological reasons for their symptoms.

On the other hand, these very same doctors recognize that many of these patients have no mental or psychological problems. In many cases, they do want to believe what these patients are telling them. This may leave doctors feeling conflicted. Do they believe what the patient is telling them, or do they believe what science is saying with the physical examination, and various medical tests that, for all practical purposes, are negative? What should be done with a patient who exhibits a variety of symptoms, which may range from humdrum to exotic, but for whom no test can find anything wrong? It should be noted that a lack of positive medical tests alone is not uncommon for some types of health problems. Headaches and back pain often lack positive findings on medical tests. Yet these problems can often be successfully resolved or controlled with exercise, stretching, medication, spinal adjustment or physical therapy.

Several options are available to the physician. The doctor can continue to treat these patients, but this is eventually demoralizing to the doctor due to the constant failure of the patients to show significant progress. Even if the patient is happy with the doctor's effort, the doctor may question why ongoing treatments should continue with so little benefit. Many doctors also have the misguided idea that they may be rewarding emotional neediness with the diagnosis and treatment of these conditions.[1]

Referral of the patient to another doctor is a reasonable option, but is also fraught with problems. Many patients feel abandoned when this is done, especially when they have already been to other specialists who have been of no help. In addition, when the specialist has failed, these patients often come back anyway. Ongoing referral by the primary care physician may also feel unethical in an over-burdened health care system already suffering from spiraling costs. Even doctors who are considered good in almost every other respect may eventually resent or refuse to treat the patients who have these conditions.

Understanding Both Points of View

I believe it is worthwhile to recognize that having a nonplus condition is not only difficult for the people suffering with these conditions; it is also confusing for the doctors treating them. This may help you understand some doctor's attitudes of frustration, apathy or even blame when you do seek medical attention. Most physicians are doing the very best they can with disorders that make little or no sense given their current level of understanding. No matter how much a doctor wants to believe that the patient is actually suffering from physical causes, science and in some ways even ethical considerations may tell her to label the patient as psychosomatic, depressed, or needy. I am not saying all doctors or even most doctors feel this way, but I do feel that most doctors have felt this way from time to time. I know I have.

As easy as it is to blame emotional or psychological problems as being the cause of these conditions, this is not logical or scientific in most cases. Studies have pointed out that while some people with nonplus conditions do experience underlying mood disorders, they do not do so at a greater rate than those suffering from other chronic illnesses.[2] Other studies have shown that medical research indicating that chronic fatigue is the result of psychiatric illnesses is based on flawed assumptions.[3] If you are seeing a doctor who does not believe that your symptoms are due to a true physical problem, you should consider seeing another doctor.

In spite of the controversy and confusion surrounding these syndromes there has been progress. Acknowledging groups of symptoms that commonly go together and giving them a name as has been done with the terms chronic fatigue, fibromyalgia, interstitial cystitis, irritable bowel syndrome, chemical sensitivity and others is a positive step. Most of these conditions are now recognized by authoritative organizations such as the Centers for Disease Control and the American College of Rheumatology. Nevertheless, for the average practicing physician to feel more confident about diagnosing and treating the nonplus conditions, more information is needed on their most basic and essential facts. It is these facts that will allow doctors to see the patterns and relationships that will make the nonplus conditions understandable. This is no less true for the person who is suffering with a nonplus condition and is searching for a way to make sense of what is happening.

If guaifenesin helps us to make sense of the nonplus conditions, it would not be the first time that an effective treatment helps us to more fully understand conditions that were previously a mystery. Before the discovery of cortisone through a series of fortuitous and coincidental events, there was no knowledge that upwards of 200 different illnesses, many arthritic in nature, were connected by a process called inflammation.[4]

One of the most common questions I receive from patients is, "Do my symptoms make sense?" People want to feel that their problems have some logical explanation. I hope that this book will enable people with a nonplus condition and the doctors treating them to finally see that yes, their symptoms do follow a pattern and they do make sense. There are still a great many important questions to be answered about fibromyalgia, chronic fatigue, irritable bowel, multiple chemical sensitivity and all of the conditions that I refer to as the nonplus conditions, but with the information in this book readers will possess a more complete understanding and a truly effective treatment for these difficult health problems.

1

Understanding fibromyalgia, chronic fatigue, irritable bowel and the other nonplus conditions

I vaguely remember hearing about fibromyalgia, chronic fatigue, and chemical sensitivities when I was still in college, although I am not sure if these were the names used at that time. Within my first several years of practice, I once again started hearing these terms, this time from my own patients. Most of these patients were hungry for more information, but had learned from years of seeing doctors that the majority of them, like me, knew little or nothing about these conditions. As a result, these patients were eager to share with me their understanding of fibromyalgia, chronic fatigue and similar conditions that they were experiencing with the hope that it would spark in me a desire to learn more. These patients would tell me about their symptoms and the many doctors and specialists they had seen who were either unwilling to treat them because of the prejudice surrounding these conditions or were unable to provide anything more than temporary relief. I found myself baffled by their symptoms, but also intrigued that so many apparently common conditions lacked recognition and effective treatments. This was in stark contrast to the rapid advances of health care with other health problems from AIDS to heart disease.

It was from these persistent, pioneering patients that I received my initial education regarding the difficult-to-diagnose-and-treat problems that I now refer to as the nonplus conditions. I use the term nonplus since these conditions have most doctors "nonplused" or baffled. Fibromyalgia, irritable bowel and chronic fatigue are now the most commonly known conditions in this group and recognition from physicians has increased gradually since the 1980's when many of these conditions began to be discussed by greater numbers of people. In spite of increased awareness, discussion and research on these conditions, the difficulties in understanding what they are and how to effectively treat them remain largely unchanged. In fact, all of the closely related health problems that make up the nonplus conditions, Ehlers-Danlos Syndrome, interstitial cystitis, multiple chemical sensitivity, neurally mediated hypotension, restless legs, and vulvodynia as well as irritable bowel, chronic fatigue and fibromyalgia remain medical enigmas. I believe that the ongoing confusion regarding these conditions stems partly from the fact that each conditions is usually studied independently. This prevents a more complete picture of these conditions from being seen. An umbrella term such as nonplus will help the larger picture to become more obvious with its tacit acknowledgement of the close relationships of these 10 conditions.

The term nonplus is also useful because it eliminates the need to individually list all ten conditions that frequently occur together and often respond to the same nonprescription medication. In addition, nonplus is a word with meanings that capture the essence of how these conditions often feel to the people who suffer from them, as well as the experience of the doctors who have patients with them. According to Webster's New Collegiate Dictionary, the word nonplus has two meanings, both of which are applicable when used to name confusing and frustrating conditions. As a noun, it can mean: "a state of bafflement or perplexity" and as a verb transitive: "to cause to be at a loss as to what to say, think, or do."[1] The similarities and interrelated nature of the nonplus conditions are covered in greater detail in chapter 4.

During my years in practice I have gradually become more and more determined to find effective treatments for the nonplus conditions because a significant number of my patients have one or more of them. The longer I practiced, the more I was able to recognize these conditions in my patients and to my astonishment, in myself as well. My own deteriorating health, due to several of these conditions, was another major motivator behind a seemingly endless search for answers. In the past 24 years, I have gradually learned more about how to manage these conditions with lifestyle changes, treating individual symptoms, and by finding and treating unrelated health problems that contribute additional symptoms. I was always mindful, however, that managing the pain and malfunction caused by the nonplus conditions was not the same as an effective treatment that addressed the underlying cause of these problems and that could create long-lasting relief of all associated symptoms.

When attempting to help people with these conditions, I was open to a wide range of possible treatments and suggestions from my patients. I tried many different approaches including supplements, diets, ways to exercise, stress management and physical medicine procedures such as chiropractic and physical therapy. After 19 years in practice I learned about guaifenesin (gwi-FEN-e-sin), a safe and inexpensive nonprescription medication based on the herb guaiac from the Guaiacum tree. Because guaifenesin is almost devoid of side effects and is readily available, I began using it personally to see if it would help me with my nonplus symptoms. This was not because I had any particular belief in guaifenesin, but because I tried almost everything that claimed to be of help and appeared to be even remotely reasonable.

I was pleasantly surprised when I began to experience some significant improvements within a month. Because of my success, I soon began helping my patients who suffered with one or more of the nonplus conditions use guaifenesin, and I was equally surprised when most of them also improved. Since then, I have continued to help hundreds of patients use guaifenesin. Most have seen significant, long-lasting, and ongoing improvements. Some now even feel they have recovered completely, something I had never seen prior to using guaifenesin.

My initial years of using guaifenesin on patients required a steep learning curve on what it takes to get optimal results. There are several important steps (the guaifenesin protocol) that need to be followed, and my office was carefully guiding each patient through these steps. Unfortunately, I found another largely unrecognized obstacle that could prevent anyone using guaifenesin from getting results. The problem was brands of extended-release guaifenesin that were ineffective. In the fall of 2000, I began to see indications that patients using some brands of extended release guaifenesin were consistently having difficulty finding a dose of guaifenesin that gave relief. Because of this, I had my patients use only guaifenesin that I knew to be effective.

The FDA has now largely remedied the problem. Unfortunately, before it was resolved, it is likely that thousands of individuals who used poorly manufactured extended-release guaifenesin did not improve and gave up on using it to treat fibromyalgia and the rest of the nonplus conditions. The reason I bring this topic up is so that people who may have used extended-release guaifenesin in the past will be aware that this could have been the reason for a lack of results. Thankfully, there have been many thousands of people worldwide who have used guaifenesin that was effective and have benefited from its use.

An important side note is that all guaifenesin products that have registered and listed their product with the FDA and have followed the labeling and ingredient requirements now have equal standing with the FDA. No legally sold guaifenesin has a higher approval status with the FDA than another.[2]

The names of the individual nonplus conditions do not indicate that these conditions are related. Nevertheless, all of them have much more in common than it appears from their names alone. Doctors, researchers, and textbooks that are knowledgeable in the individual nonplus conditions have noticed that several of these conditions frequently occur together and that the symptoms of these disorders overlap. When a person has several nonplus conditions, it can be difficult to tell where the symptoms of one condition end and the symptoms of another condition begin. The idea that fibromyalgia, chronic fatigue, irritable bowel, chemical sensitivities, and some of the other nonplus conditions are somehow related has been discussed for decades. *Kelley's Rheumatology* states, "The differences between the syndromes characterized by chronic pain and fatigue are more semantic than real, and the demarcations that have been established to separate these conditions are largely historical and artificial."[3]

I have identified specific characteristics that highlight the similarities shared by the different nonplus conditions. The four primary characteristics are:

1. Each of these conditions is more likely to occur with other nonplus conditions than they are to occur alone. In addition, the conditions share many of the same symptoms.
2. Difficulty of diagnosis is due to a lack of signs or positive medical tests that can positively identify them and little if any understanding of the underlying cause.
3. A lack of effective, long-lasting treatments that can improve all related symptoms associated with these conditions.
4. Guaifenesin gradually improves, and in many cases, eventually eliminates the symptoms of these conditions.

Despite some acknowledgement that the individual nonplus conditions share many common traits and possibly a common cause, there continues to be confusion and controversy associated with all of the nonplus conditions. This controversy involves almost everything about these conditions including the possible cause or causes, the most effective treatments and even whether, in fact, these conditions do exist. As is often the case in medicine, when a health problem is not understood, the condition may be ignored or the blame put upon the patient for causing or inventing it. For decades, many of the nonplus conditions have been blamed upon depression, a need for attention, stress, type A personality, and other similar explanations.

The third edition of *Practical Rheumatology* from 2004, a textbook for physicians who specialize in rheumatology, directly addresses the difficulties medicine has had in accepting fibromyalgia. In discussing the history of fibromyalgia, this book states, "fibrositis, as it was then called, was considered by some to be a common cause of muscular pain, by others to be a manifestation of 'tension' or 'psychogenic rheumatism' and by the rheumatology community in general to be a nonentity."[4] It can be argued that all of the nonplus conditions have been ignored, avoided, or denigrated in a similar way at some point in the past.

Fortunately for patients, all the nonplus conditions are now ridiculed or ignored less frequently. In medical textbooks, most of these conditions are recognized for what they actually are: baffling and difficult to treat clusters of characteristic symptoms that have an unknown cause. In this way the nonplus conditions are not unlike many other illnesses, from lupus erythematosus to multiple sclerosis. It is unfortunate that while many treating physicians are becoming more aware and tolerant of these conditions, some doctors still view them as an irritation in their practice that will not go away.

This controversy has continued over the decades primarily because of the difficulties that the nonplus conditions present when attempting to study or treat them. The three primary reasons that the nonplus conditions persist in being controversial are:

1. The cause of the nonplus conditions remains unknown. Many theories have been proposed, but none are proven.
2. The nonplus conditions are difficult to diagnose. They do not usually signal their existence in the form of signs, (i.e., elevated temperature, dilated pupils, edema, rash), nor do routine diagnostic tests such as x-rays, ultrasound, or blood tests identify them.
3. Symptoms resulting from the nonplus conditions rarely respond to treatment, can number in the dozens, and vary widely in their intensity and frequency. In addition, the number of active symptoms may change from week to week in some people or remain stable for years in other people.

In other words, the nonplus conditions are confusing because it is hard to know when a person has one of them since there are no tests that can tell doctors when a nonplus condition is present. In addition, there is no obvious cause, symptoms may come and go without reason and, up to now, no effective treatment is available. This almost total lack of information creates a Catch-22 situation. Without the existence of signs or positive medical tests, doctors are not sure of the diagnosis, leaving them up in the air about what condition to treat. If they decide to just treat individual symptoms, the lack of long-lasting improvement results leaves them frustrated. With no positive tests and little or no response to symptom treatment, they are unsure how to proceed. Due to the general lack of treatment results, some doctors are not even sure if they should continue with any treatment.

It is easy to see how devastating these difficulties can be for a person if we consider the effects of only one nonplus condition. For example, let us imagine a person with irritable bowel and how it alone can affect their life. Irritable bowel may cause one or all of the following symptoms: nausea, bloating, indigestion, constipation, diarrhea and abdominal cramping among others. These symptoms may vary greatly from week to week or even day to day. Eating meals may feel like Russian roulette since there is no way for a person to know how their body will react. Will they simply be able to enjoy a meal or will they suffer for hours or days later? When a doctor is consulted, many tests will eventually be preformed. If the problem is actually irritable bowel, however, the medical tests are negative.

What are this person and the doctor to do if no evidence of malfunction, infection, cancer, ulcer, or even an elevated temperature is found? What is this person to do if after months or even years of ongoing tests, the pain and malfunction remains, but nothing is found amiss? Worse yet, what if a variety of medications, lifestyle changes, supplements, and alternative treatments give only occasional or no relief? Most often, the individuals and their doctors are at a loss as to what to think or do. They are nonplused. This gives an idea of how it feels to have a nonplus condition.

The lack of signs and diagnostic tests are somewhat helpful by telling doctors what conditions a person does not have. Thus, it is usually only after no other cause for a patient's symptom can be found that a nonplus condition is diagnosed. However, the nonplus conditions are not merely a diagnosis of exclusion, they must also be diagnosed by their own characteristic features. Nevertheless, ruling out other conditions should be done before the nonplus conditions are diagnosed.

For example, when a person is experiencing exhaustion or fatigue, there are many possible reasons. A person could be over-worked, lack sleep, have inadequate nutrition, be depressed, or have endocrine problems. When all these and more have been considered and ruled out, chronic fatigue may be considered. Nonplus conditions can also exist alongside any other condition such as heart or thyroid problems and cause considerable confusion as to why a person is not responding to standard care for these conventional conditions.

The nonplus conditions have many similarities, but when it comes to diagnosis, fibromyalgia and chronic fatigue pose a greater level of difficulty than the other nonplus conditions. This is due to fibromyalgia and chronic fatigue having such a wide variety of possible symptoms, resulting in a great many health issues to rule out. Symptoms like pain all over, fatigue, mental sluggishness, depression, nonrestful sleep, rapid heartbeat, weakened immune system, sinus problems, brittle nails, jaw pain, and itching do not follow a pattern. It may be necessary to rule out many different illnesses that involve all of the different body systems. The ruling-out process usually includes a physical examination, patient history, and possibly blood work, x-rays, and other tests, depending upon the symptoms a person has and the doctor's area of expertise.

Because of this, it is not uncommon for it to take five or more years for a person with fibromyalgia or chronic fatigue to be accurately diagnosed. In contrast, the urinary tract symptoms and pelvic pain that occur with interstitial cystitis may be as debilitating to the patient as fibromyalgia, but to a doctor, the process of ruling out all possible causes of pelvic pain is less complex and time consuming since the symptoms are generally confined to one area of the body.

Despite much research to the contrary, a surprising number of doctors still consider some of the nonplus conditions to be "junk diagnoses." The implication is that some doctors use these terms when they do not know what else to call a patient's symptoms. In my practice, I see little evidence that most doctors are actually doing this indicating that the junk diagnosis moniker is largely unfounded. Actually, I believe that the opposite is true. Due to ignorance or bias regarding the nonplus conditions, these conditions are under-diagnosed. I see considerably more patients who have an undiagnosed nonplus condition than I see patients who are improperly diagnosed as having a nonplus condition. The junk diagnoses that I most often encounter are terms like arthritis, stress, and depression to explain symptoms of pain, fatigue, difficulty sleeping or digestive problems. In addition, this term "junk diagnosis" when used for nonplus conditions is unfair, because it ultimately puts a negative label on the patient for having a condition that our health care system has yet to solve.

There are still some physicians who believe the nonplus conditions are due to depression or stress. In the absence of scientific proof, bewildering chronic illnesses may be treated as psychological problems. Peptic ulcers were blamed on personality and chronic anxiety for more than 25 years. In the 1980's, Barry Marshall discovered a bacteria, H. pylori, and proved that peptic ulcers were in large part due to a bacterial infection, not dietary or emotional reasons.[5] Multiple sclerosis was similarly blamed by some on stress until imaging technology could show that MS is based on abnormalities of the nervous system and has a physical cause.[6] Studies on the incidence of identifiable mood disorders such as depression and anxiety in individuals with fibromyalgia compared to other chronic medical conditions show little difference.[7] Some people have pointed out that the depression which occurs with chronic illnesses lacking medical acceptance, as is the case with the nonplus conditions, can be better described as demoralization.[8]

Until a cause is found or testing can make a positive identification, the nonplus conditions are simply sets of characteristic symptoms of unknown origin that have been given a name. In most cases the name of the condition describes its primary symptom. For example, the name chronic fatigue leaves no doubt as to the primary symptom of this malady even though there are dozens of additional symptoms that are often associated with it. Some of the nonplus conditions have only one symptom or are limited to just one area of the body. This may also be reflected in its name. Restless legs syndrome, for example, involves an irresistible urge to frequently move the legs.

As previously discussed, treatment is another area of difficulty for those suffering from a nonplus condition. Even the most basic symptoms associated with them are notoriously difficult to treat. Sore muscles, pain, fatigue, and digestive distress usually have concrete causes and specific treatments. When the cause of these and other symptoms is due to nonplus conditions, there may not be any treatment that gives even temporary relief. The inability to find effective treatments adds considerably to the confusion and frustration surrounding all of the nonplus conditions. This is yet another reason why some doctors are reluctant to treat them. Because of a long history of resistance to treatment, people may believe that effective treatment is impossible. After trying dozens of possible treatments over a period of more than 15 years, I was also skeptical of any product or approach that claimed to create long-term improvement. Using guaifenesin on hundreds of patients has changed my mind, allowing me to see that a helpful long-term treatment is possible for most people.

Using guaifenesin to treat the nonplus conditions is still relatively unknown. This is in large part because the individual nonplus conditions are little known and poorly defined conditions to many physicians. For physicians who are aware of and treat one or more of the nonplus conditions, getting their attention on an obscure treatment for confusing conditions is not easy. For the average person looking for help, the marketplace is filled with products whose claims are overblown or completely inaccurate. This has resulted in people and physicians becoming suspicious of any treatment for these conditions. Third, and possibly most importantly, success when using guaifenesin is dependent upon using it in a carefully prescribed manner. Simply taking an arbitrary amount of guaifenesin on a daily basis is unlikely to produce symptomatic improvements.

People diagnosed with nonplus conditions are often told by well-meaning physicians that they must learn to live with these health problems. Fortunately, this is no longer the case for most individuals. With the proper use of guaifenesin the chances of recovery are excellent. Although guaifenesin is best known for treating fibromyalgia, I would like to emphasize that all of the nonplus conditions are treated equally effectively with guaifenesin.

2

Treating the Nonplus Conditions

Fibromyalgia and chronic fatigue are the best known of the nonplus conditions. Because of the great number and wide range of possible symptoms, they are also more controversial than the other nonplus conditions with the possible exception of multiple chemical sensitivity. Multiple chemical sensitivity has unique features that make it especially difficult to study and treat. Having multiple chemical sensitivities can result in any of the symptoms that occur with nonplus conditions, but the symptoms are associated with exposure to chemicals or fumes common in every day living and which are usually considered harmless.

The extent of symptoms common to these three conditions adds considerably to the difficulty in understanding, recognizing, and treating them. Not everyone with fibromyalgia, chronic fatigue and multiple chemical sensitivities experiences dozens of symptoms; but for those who do, treating all of these different symptoms is difficult. Individuals and their doctors can easily feel overwhelmed with this seemingly impossible task. This is especially true because the symptoms of the nonplus conditions change frequently and typically respond only slightly, if at all, to treatment.

The remaining nonplus conditions, irritable bowel syndrome, Ehlers-

Danlos Syndrome, immune dysfunction syndrome, interstitial cystitis, neurally mediated hypotension, restless legs syndrome and vulvodynia have fewer possible symptoms and the symptoms are generally associated with one system or part of the body. The symptoms of these conditions, although fewer in number and slightly more predictable in nature, are just as difficult to treat as the symptoms of fibromyalgia, chronic fatigue and multiple chemical sensitivity.

How do treatments help?

There are a great many products claiming that they are helpful in treating nonplus conditions, especially for the better known conditions of chronic fatigue and fibromyalgia. Many books, companies, and websites promote everything from vitamins and hormones to exercises and bed mattresses as being helpful. Fortunately, some of these approaches do help to control a few symptoms in some people. What I have not seen is a thoughtful discussion on what it is that these treatments are actually doing. Different types of treatments manage symptoms in different ways. A basic understanding of how approaches differ can lead to more effective symptom management.

Currently, treatment for the nonplus conditions involves three major approaches:

1. Lifestyle and body optimization. This approach helps people to make the most of a body that does not always work well. Examples of this approach would include eating a healthy balanced diet, taking supplements, using relaxation techniques and getting regular exercise and sleep. Lifestyle may have to be altered in some ways to manage symptoms, such as reducing activities to prevent exhaustion, or avoiding activities that cause pain.
2. Treating individual symptoms. This could include an ice bag on the neck, spinal manipulation, massage, or taking medications for pain and other symptoms.
3. Treating unrelated and sometimes overlooked conditions that are unknowingly contributing to symptoms caused by the nonplus conditions. Common examples include thyroid conditions, yeast

infections, spinal misalignments, hormone imbalance, reactive hypoglycemia, and trigger points.

These treatments are indirect treatments that help to manage symptoms but do little or nothing to influence the mechanism behind the nonplus conditions. All of the current treatments that I know of, except for guaifenesin, treat the nonplus conditions in one of the three ways just discussed. All of these approaches are valid and should be used when appropriate especially when pain, fatigue, or other symptoms are making life difficult.

These three therapeutic approaches are helpful but incomplete. I, like other individuals, have been grateful for the help that they have given, but have also been disappointed by their shortcomings. A simple but illustrative example may help to make my point more clear. If a person had a thorn in their foot, they could use the above therapeutic approaches to some advantage. Lifestyle could be of help by promoting healing with the use of healthy food, vitamins, and positive thinking. Crutches are another lifestyle change that would help to prevent irritation to the foot in the area where the thorn was inserted. Controlling symptoms could be accomplished with painkillers and anti-inflammatory medications or supplements that have a similar effect. Of course we would want to correct any other problems with the foot that was contributing to foot problems such as gout, ingrown toe nails and athlete's foot.

Many of these treatments, however, will prove to be unnecessary if we use a fourth treatment approach.

4. Treating the underlying cause.

Pulling the thorn out of the foot would directly treat the cause of the problem and if done soon enough would likely make many of the other treatments just discussed unnecessary or at least secondary.

Until guaifenesin, there was nothing available to directly treat the nonplus conditions. A treatment that addresses the underlying cause should give long-lasting relief for all symptoms. In my experience and that of other physicians and thousands of individuals, only guaifenesin is often able to improve and eventually resolve all symptoms caused by the nonplus conditions for people who use it correctly. This indicates that in some way guaifenesin is directly treating a core part of these problems and not simply temporarily covering up or managing symptoms. Because guaifenesin therapy directly addresses the underlying mechanism responsible for causing the nonplus conditions it is fundamentally different from the other three types of indirect treatments.

Treating Cause VS Understanding Cause

Since the cause or causes of the nonplus conditions are still unknown or at least hotly debated, a reasonable question is, "How is it possible to treat the cause when the mechanism creating these health problems remains a mystery?

Every time a person eats enough of a particular vitamin or mineral to prevent a nutritional deficiency disease, we can say that in a very real way they are treating or preventing health problems such as anemia, scurvy, and osteoporosis. Thankfully, there is no need to understand the inner workings of biochemistry and human physiology in order for different nutrients to do their jobs. All that is required is that the body's nutritional needs be met; whether this is by accident or intention is unimportant to the body.

When it comes to doctors treating diseases, most people believe that a complete understanding of a disease is necessary before an effective treatment is found. Although this belief sounds reasonable, in fact, treatments are often found by trial and error or by chance observation long before other important facts, such as the cause of the disease, are known.

There are many facts to learn before a general understanding of a disease occurs. Some of the important facts to know are: what is the cause or causes of a particular condition, what are the risk factors for acquiring the condition, what are the signs or symptoms, is there a way to prevent it, how does the condition progress, what are effective treatments if any, how do treatments work and so on. In most cases, these facts are discovered gradually over a period of many years and there is no particular order in which the different pieces of the disease puzzle are learned. If a beneficial treatment is found before all of the other facts are known, the treatment itself becomes an important piece of information providing doctors and researchers with another clue about the nature of the condition.

For many decades, up to and through the 1980's, stomach ulcers were blamed on stress and spicy food. The fallacy of this belief became clear due to the effectiveness of an unlikely treatment using antibiotics and championed by only a handful of doctors. The treatment and understanding of stomach ulcers is now forever changed, not just because the effectiveness of this treatment, but also because it disproved a longstanding and erroneous theory regarding the cause of stomach ulcers. The treatment in this case was an indispensable clue about the true nature and cause of the condition. Many other important treatments in the fields of rheumatology, infectious diseases, and mental health came about before all of the facts were known about a particular condition.

The above example shows us that it is not necessary for us to understand everything about the nonplus conditions for an effective treatment to exist. Although guaifenesin appears to be altering some aspect of the underlying cause of the nonplus conditions, it is not correcting the cause. When a person stops guaifenesin, the symptoms that were eliminated or reduced usually begin to return. As the cause or causes of the nonplus conditions are believed to be genetic, eliminating them is unlikely unless or until gene therapy is developed.

What is guaifenesin?

Guaifenesin is a safe and inexpensive nonprescription compound. It does not affect or react with any other prescription or nonprescription drug.[1] A related compound, guaiac, was derived from the guaiacum tree in the 1500s and used to treat rheumatic complaints until the early 1800s.[2] Guaifenesin is the modern manufactured version of guaiac and is known to thin mucus secretions and make coughs more productive. Because of this, it is in cough and cold preparations. Like many medications, however, guaifenesin has more than one effect and is able to treat several types of health problems. When used to treat the nonplus conditions, guaifenesin must be combined with several additional therapeutic steps, sometimes called the guaifenesin protocol, in order to be effective. These steps are briefly reviewed at the beginning of this book in The Guaifenesin Guide Quick Reference and are discussed at length in chapters 7, 8 and 9.

The significance of having a treatment like guaifenesin that addresses the underlying cause resulting in the improvement of all related symptoms is hard to overstate. In patients with dozens of symptoms caused by one or more of the nonplus conditions, managing every symptom is difficult. Every day in my practice, I now see patients who are greatly improved as a result of using guaifenesin, but it was not always this way. Finding effective treatments for the various nonplus conditions had been an ongoing goal of mine since I started treating patients in 1982. I believed that there must be some logical explanation or an overlooked aspect that would explain why various symptoms would mysteriously appear, and persist in spite of all treatments conventional and alternative.

Traditional treatments not addressing cause

My efforts at finding solutions were actually spurred on by what appeared to be the nonsensical results I saw when treating my patients. I wanted to understand why many people who did not have a nonplus condition could often give little thought to good health practices, but would nevertheless quickly respond to treatment for common symptoms like fatigue or back pain. On the other hand, people with nonplus conditions who conscientiously followed healthy lifestyles would often have difficulty responding to any treatment.

Over time I realized that if lifestyle were the sole determinate of one's health, then many of my most difficult and nonresponsive patients should be some of the healthiest people on the planet because of their commitment to good health practices such as diet, exercise, regular sleep and stress management. For millions of people with nonplus conditions, however, their commitment to an optimal lifestyle does not lead to buoyant health, merely survival. In many cases, when a person has a nonplus condition, any deviation from their carefully scripted routine of diet, supplements, activity avoidance, rest or other activities quickly results in increased pain and other problems.

This issue of having to live with such attention to detail and still suffering from considerable pain, fatigue or other symptoms is something that many of my patients complain about as being maddening and unfair. Eventually, most people come to recognize that optimizing a sick body with special care is not the same as treating the underlying problem that is causing the malfunction. As a result, people with the nonplus conditions are always looking for something that provides long-term relief for all symptoms.

An integral part of my practice is to address the cause of my patient's problems whenever possible, and to treat symptoms only when necessary. However, I grew increasingly frustrated as I realized that no treatments seemed to address the cause of the health problems I now call the nonplus conditions. Even treating the symptoms of these conditions was difficult and seldom rewarded with ideal results. Partly out of a desire to improve my own deteriorating health, I remained open to new solutions and I spent many years looking for all types of imbalances and deficiencies. I tried what seemed like an endless variety of dietary recommendations, nutritional supplements, exercises, physical medicine procedures, stretches, magnets, and mental relaxation techniques to name a few.

I also followed the progress of my patients with one or more of the nonplus conditions who were seeing other physicians. These doctors used medications, trigger point injections, amalgam removal from teeth, psychological counseling, nutritional supplements, physical therapies, chiropractic techniques, acupuncture along with other oriental therapies and herbs. No matter how many specialists were seen or treatments used, my patients reported that the majority of their symptoms persisted with little if any long-term improvement.

Maximizing the benefit of conventional treatments

All this effort did pay off in small ways, and as the years went by I was able to better recognize—and to a certain extent treat—the different nonplus conditions, particularly fibromyalgia, chronic fatigue, irritable bowel and multiple chemical sensitivities. I did not know much about the other nonplus conditions until after I started using guaifenesin.

Patients would sometimes come to see me specifically because they had heard that I was good at helping fibromyalgia, etc. I would explain that I might be able to help, but not because I could treat these conditions directly (this was before I started using guaifenesin). What I could do was acknowledge their illness and support them by helping them to find and resolve contributing conditions; suggest lifestyle improvements; and help them to manage at least some of their pain or other problems by treating individual symptoms. I learned that by using all three of these treatment approaches that I had available at the time, I could have some success in treating patients with nonplus conditions. I would continue working with these patients until a variety of treatments were tried or considered for every symptom.

With general symptoms such as joint, muscle, and back pain, I would often find and treat two, three, or more problems that were contributing to this. For example, a person with fibromyalgia who had low back pain might also have a psoas muscle strain, lumbar vertebra subluxations, foot pronation requiring orthotics, and sacroiliac ligament strain. Once these problems were corrected, some people would have their low back pain completely resolved. This indicated that fibromyalgia or the other nonplus conditions were not the cause of low back pain in this patient, even if fibromyalgia was the cause of pain in other areas. Other patients might only have partial improvement after these types of problems were corrected, indicating that fibromyalgia was at least partially responsible for their low back pain. A third group of patients with fibromyalgia and low back pain might not have any structural or muscular issues whatsoever. In this case, fibromyalgia might be the sole cause of the low back pain.

Nonplus conditions, a common cause of persistent symptoms

When commonly recognized medical conditions are not present, persistent discomfort or fatigue is not always due to fibromyalgia, chronic fatigue, and the other nonplus conditions. Several other conditions that are less recognized, or are especially difficult to diagnose can also be responsible for persistent symptoms. A few of the possible examples are permanent damage due to an injury, congenital defects, Lyme Disease and others. Even when these other issues are considered, I have found that in my practice, the most common reason for ongoing problems in a patient that are resistant to treatment was because of a nonplus condition. This leads me to believe that the nonplus conditions occur much more frequently than is currently acknowledged. Leonard Jason, Ph.D. from DePaul University led a study on chronic fatigue involving more than 18,000 people. From the findings of this study, it appears chronic fatigue is many times more common than previously believed.[3] Although this study was only on chronic fatigue, I believe that the same can be said for most of the other nonplus conditions as well.

Confusion about what condition is being treated

Several situations can arise that can confuse people into thinking that they have successfully treated a nonplus condition when in reality, they have not. This occurs when: [1] A person is diagnosed as having a nonplus condition when in reality they do not, or [2] A person actually has a nonplus condition, but has other conditions as well which are aggravating the symptoms from the nonplus conditions.

For example, a person suffers from cramping and diarrhea following a course of antibiotics. These digestive symptoms may persist for month after month or even years. Medical tests show no evidence of disease so the eventual diagnosis becomes irritable bowel syndrome. Finally, possibly years later, someone recommends this person take a probiotic supplement such as lactobacilli acidophilus. Because of this supplement, all symptoms clear. This person and their doctor may now wrongly believe that lactobacillus acidophilus is a treatment for irritable bowel syndrome. This would be an inaccurate conclusion since this person never actually had irritable bowel syndrome. The antibiotic that was taken years before to treat an infection killed some of the beneficial bacteria that normally inhabit the colon. The absence of these "good bacteria" caused what is called an intestinal dysbiosis, which in turn creates problems in the digestive tract such as diarrhea, bloating, nausea, and gas. It is situations like this that can lead people to wrongly believe that they have treated and resolved a nonplus condition when they have actually treated an unrelated health problem which happens to cause similar symptoms.

A variation on this is when an undiscovered health problem is contributing to symptoms already present because of the nonplus conditions. This situation was already discussed previously with the example of finding several factors contributing to low back pain. Another example could be if a person has both irritable bowel syndrome and an intestinal dysbiosis. When a probiotic supplement is taken, some of the symptoms are decreased or eliminated. This improvement occurred because the intestinal dysbiosis was treated, not because probiotics are therapeutic for irritable bowel. Not everyone with irritable bowel has a dysbiosis and certainly, most people with a dysbiosis do not have irritable bowel. Partial improvement of symptoms under these circumstances may once again result in a person and their physician erroneously believing that a specific treatment is helpful for or resolves irritable bowel.

Misunderstandings like these can occur with many different nutrients or therapies commonly used on individuals with nonplus conditions. A person low in magnesium may experience decreased energy levels, constipation, muscle cramps, headaches, and chest pain, regardless of whether any other condition is present including a nonplus condition. If a product with enough magnesium is taken, all of these symptoms may improve or be eliminated completely. When this type of relief occurs in a person who does have fibromyalgia, irritable bowel, or chronic fatigue, it may be wrongly concluded that magnesium is an actual treatment for these conditions. While I agree that magnesium should be considered whenever the symptoms of a magnesium deficiency are present, or if tests reveal a magnesium deficiency, I do not believe that magnesium deficiency is the cause or even a cause of any of the nonplus conditions. Magnesium will help a person with one of the nonplus conditions only if they are magnesium deficient. This is no different than a B-12, iron, or iodine deficiency. Eliminating nutritional deficiencies can eliminate certain symptoms in anyone, with or without a nonplus condition.

Nutritional deficiencies are just one type of health problem that can contribute to the symptoms already being caused by nonplus conditions. There are many other examples of symptoms having more than one cause. Shoulder blade pain frequently occurs with fibromyalgia; however, there are at least four other common causes for this pain. Biliary stasis (gallbladder problems), trigger points, thoracic subluxation, and a misaligned first rib can all cause or contribute to this pain. It is not uncommon to find several of these imbalances in one person. Best results will be achieved when all contributing factors are diagnosed and treated.

Why does it matter if magnesium or eliminating a yeast infection is credited as being an effective treatment for a nonplus condition? I believe it does matter because these types of myths contribute to confusion surrounding the nonplus conditions. It is partly because of these types of misunderstandings that there are so many inaccurate claims regarding treatments for nonplus conditions. This inaccurate information is why people are inclined to ignore treatment that purports to be helpful for nonplus conditions.

Long-term treatment for all symptoms

As difficult as diagnosing the nonplus conditions is, treating them is even more difficult. Tens of thousands of individuals are properly diagnosed, but few have recovered. In many cases of people who believe that they have recovered, the symptoms have actually switched from one nonplus condition to another. In my practice I frequently see patients who have a variety of problems such as bladder pain and urgency in the absence of infection (interstitial cystitis), non-restful sleep, blurred vision, difficulty thinking, and feeling light headed at times when in an upright position (neurally mediated hypotension). When I ask these patients if they have heard of fibromyalgia or chronic fatigue, a frequent response is, "Yes, I used to have that but I got rid of it with vitamins, organic food, yoga, etc". Few of these patients realize that their current symptoms are from the same source as their previous symptoms of chronic fatigue.

It has been my experience that even the doctor who is knowledgeable enough to accurately diagnose these conditions is not able to provide effective and long-lasting treatments, unless guaifenesin is used. In my pre-guaifenesin practice, I struggled with the realities of limited results whenever I treated anyone with a nonplus condition. I continued reading and taking classes to find out more about these problems. Year after year, I listened as hundreds of my patients with nonplus conditions told me about their previous doctors' approaches and how most treatments gave limited, if any, relief. Dozens of patients told me how insulted they were when a doctor told them that nothing was wrong and that they should just "get over it." Others were told by doctors that they were depressed or sleep deprived, but found that antidepressants or sleep medications helped only a few if any symptoms. Some doctors refused to even attempt to treat fibromyalgia and chronic fatigue, stating that nothing could be done.

These conversations with my patients showed me that the different nonplus conditions were incredibly difficult to treat, and that I was not the only one having trouble finding effective treatments. After years of actively pursuing answers but finding nothing that actually treated these problems in my patients or myself, I doubted an effective treatment would ever be found in my lifetime. It was not until my 19th year in practice that I came across guaifenesin as a treatment for fibromyalgia, thanks to the persistence of a patient. She brought me a book to read about using guaifenesin to treat fibromyalgia. I was less than enthused, as I thought that I had read just about everything on fibromyalgia and chronic fatigue, and I did not have the stomach for another book that told me to eat right (I already was), exercise more (that was impossible), stress less (I was already using stress management techniques), and take more vitamins and herbs (I had practically tried them all).

My patient persisted in asking my opinion of this new therapy week after week until I decided that it would be less stress to just read the book than have to continually tell her, "Sorry, I haven't gotten to it yet"—stress management in action. Upon reading the book, I was pleasantly surprised when I found out that guaifenesin was different. It did not involve more of the usual lifestyle recommendations. When taken correctly, it purportedly helped all of the related symptoms in most people. The major downside was that guaifenesin was not a quick fix. It worked slowly. Additionally, it may aggravate some symptoms temporarily as the body begins to reverse what had caused the problems in the first place. But, if it worked, I felt these were minor inconveniences. This book reiterated what I had already learned regarding reactive hypoglycemia as a common co-condition associated with nonplus conditions.

I decided I had nothing to lose by giving guaifenesin a try for my own health problems. It was my habit to personally try most every reasonable and safe treatment that I learned of. Although, after 19 years of using everything from breathing exercises to liver cleanses, I had few expectations. Nevertheless, I carefully followed each of the required therapeutic steps necessary when taking guaifenesin and went on with my life. After several weeks, some of my symptoms increased, but I was ecstatic because I could tell that guaifenesin was actually creating change as predicted.

Within three weeks, pain that I had felt in the area around my shoulder blade for more than 25 years was gone! That pain has only returned rarely, for several days at a time. Most of my other symptoms were not so easy to be rid of and have improved more slowly, with intermittent exacerbations, as is typical with guaifenesin. Nonetheless, I quickly saw that this treatment was different from anything I had ever used or that my patients had described.

Soon I was recommending guaifenesin for patients whenever they had chronic fatigue, fibromyalgia, or chemical sensitivities. Later I expanded its use to irritable bowel, and eventually saw that many other conditions responded. In the first two months of using guaifenesin in my practice, I had more success with treating these problems than I had in all my previous years in practice.

Confirmation of guaifenesin's effectiveness

A question that I constantly ask myself is, how do I know guaifenesin is working? Could I just be fooling myself? I am well aware that when initially using a new therapy it is easy for a person to believe an improvement is taking place. After about three weeks, however, it usually becomes clear whether a treatment is actually having a positive effect. With all the dozens of different approaches I used to treat nonplus conditions over the years, in all cases it soon became clear which symptoms, if any, were being helped. My expectations for guaifenesin were no greater than anything else I had tried in the past. If anything, after years of ongoing failure, I had become more skeptical of any treatment that claimed to help the nonplus conditions. On the other hand, I knew I had to be willing to try new approaches if I was ever to find a truly helpful therapy; however, I reserved judgment on every treatment until I saw results on many patients over a period of months and years.

I have been using guaifenesin in my practice since September of 2000, and I continue to see excellent results. About 10 percent of my patients achieve such good results using guaifenesin that within one or two years they feel completely recovered. In many instances, these patients want to stop taking guaifenesin since all symptoms have been eliminated. I explain to these patients that if guaifenesin is discontinued, their symptoms will likely eventually return (see Chapter 5). Unlike many medications, guaifenesin does not lose its effectiveness over time, nor does the dose need to be raised to remain effective; but discontinuing guaifenesin inevitably allows the symptoms to return. Most people do not feel completely recovered after only a year or two of use, but the longer guaifenesin is used, the greater the long-term improvement becomes. I will repeat that improvement is often interrupted by a return of one or more symptoms, and some symptoms may not improve for months or even years. During these times of temporarily increased symptoms, patience is eventually rewarded with continued improvement.

In addition to the success of many doctors and patients who have used guaifenesin, three independent sources of information lend credibility to guaifenesin's usefulness as a treatment for nonplus conditions. One source comes from a rheumatology textbook and its mention of guaiac (an herb chemically similar to guaifenesin) as an ancient treatment for rheumatism. This is discussed in detail in the next chapter.

The second source comes from individuals whom I have met in a guaifenesin support group that I have held in my office twice a month for the past several years. Local newspapers frequently print the times and dates of this *Guaifenesin Support Group for Fibromyalgia, Chronic Fatigue and Irritable Bowel*. Every year, two or three people attend the support group who discovered on their own that guaifenesin helps one of these conditions. These people report that they initially used guaifenesin for its mucus thinning properties then discovered that it also helped other symptoms. They continued using guaifenesin because of these improvements, but had no knowledge that anyone else was using guaifenesin in a similar way. They attend the support meetings out of curiosity and a desire to learn more about guaifenesin and why it helps.

An individual accidentally discovering that guaifenesin helps one or more of the nonplus conditions is extremely rare. This is because the beneficial effects of using guaifenesin for nonplus conditions is usually stopped by the presence of even small amounts of salicylates. For the average person with a nonplus condition, even brushing teeth with most toothpastes will result in salicylates entering the body in great enough quantities that guaifenesin will not be therapeutic for nonplus conditions. Another factor reducing the likelihood of an accidental discovery is that for most people there is a narrow dose at which guaifenesin works. Guaifenesin taken above or below a particular milligram amount is not likely to create obvious symptom improvement. Although only a few people are lucky enough to discover guaifenesin on their own, the fact that this does occur provides additional confirmation of guaifenesin's therapeutic value.

A third source of confirmation that guaifenesin is therapeutic for the nonplus conditions comes from my ability to accurately detect defective brands of guaifenesin. When I initially started using guaifenesin in my practice, I had roughly equal numbers of patients using the immediate-release and the sustained-release type of guaifenesin. After only several months, I noticed that the patients who were using the sustained-release guaifenesin did not get the predictable results seen in patients using immediate release guaifenesin. Sustained release guaifenesin gave varying results depending upon the brand. Results could be categorized in three ways:

1. Those who saw only very inconsistent results regardless of the dose taken.
2. Those who were getting consistent results.
3. Those who experienced no changes regardless of the dose of guaifenesin taken.

This contrasted enormously with the vast majority of people taking immediate-release guaifenesin who were getting consistent results at a relatively low dosage. When a person failed to get results with a sustained release guaifenesin, I would change them to immediate release guaifenesin or a different brand of sustained release guaifenesin. In most instances, this change in brands of guaifenesin would result in improvement for the patient. A year and a half went by and I continued to notice this difference between immediate-release and sustained release guaifenesin.

Finally, in February 2002, after I was confident of my observations, I went public with the problems I was experiencing. I believed that the sustained-release guaifenesin was not completely disintegrating. I notified the FDA as well as the primary website devoted to guaifenesin use, Guai-Support. In addition, I started my own website to notify people of my observations and suggestions.

My findings were not well received by a few in the guaifenesin community. Some people erroneously believed that because sustained release guaifenesin was (at that time, but no longer) prescription and immediate release was nonprescription, the sustained release had to be superior. However, there were a great number of people who had also noticed discrepancies in some brands of sustained-release guaifenesin and were pleased to have an explanation. A year and a half later, on October 17, 2003, the FDA confirmed my observations with a notification on their website, www.fda.gov/bbs/topics/NEWS/2003/NEW00962.html This notice explained why they were phasing out all manufacture of extended-release guaifenesin except for one brand that submitted proof of efficacy. They stated, "…certain extended-release guaifenesin products were not released in the body at the appropriate rate for an extended-release product, indicating that consumers who purchased the products may not be receiving the benefits claimed."[4]

It was only because guaifenesin does create real and longstanding improvement that I was able to tell when a guaifenesin product was effective and when it was not more than a year before the FDA came to the same conclusion.

As I continue to use guaifenesin in my practice, I see more people who feel that their lives have been returned to them. Few of these people believed that they would ever be able to find a treatment that could result in the improvement and elimination of so many of their problems.

My hope is that everyone suffering from one or more of the nonplus conditions will be able to join their ranks.

Unfortunately, there are many people who have used guaifenesin in the past but discontinued its use due to a lack of results. I have treated many such people and in many cases the problem was due to ineffective brands of sustained release guaifenesin, (a problem that has now been remedied). Now, all guaifenesin is effective for the majority of people and poor results are much more likely the result of confusion regarding salicylates or optimal dosing. In this book, I have done my best to address these problems by introducing new information that will help people to understand how to use guaifenesin in the easiest and most effective way.

Fibromyalgia, Chronic Fatigue & Irritable Bowel

3

Guaifenesin Rediscovered

In modern times, the nonplus conditions have been largely neglected by medicine. Only in the past 10 or 20 years has an understanding and acknowledgement that these conditions exist become widespread. Because of the relatively recent acceptance of the nonplus conditions, particularly chronic fatigue and fibromyalgia, it is easy to think of them as modern diseases like AIDS or this year's flu.[1] Medical writings from centuries past, however, tell us that these conditions are ancient. From these writings we can also tell that fibromyalgia had a specific and effective treatment several hundred years ago. Unfortunately, for a variety of reasons, knowledge of this effective treatment for fibromyalgia was lost sometime in the late 1700s to early 1800s.

The existence of a treatment for fibromyalgia in the distant past does not mean that it was well understood or even had a name that referred specifically to it. This is because for hundreds of years just about any health problem that caused muscular and joint pain went under the general name of rheumatism. Although muscle and ligament injuries or joint misalignments can cause muscular and joint pain, these types of problems, usually resulting from injury or physical effort, are not classified as rheumatic. Rheumatism, or rheumatic type pain is not generally associated with physical effort. We now know that the most common reason for chronic rheumatic type symptoms are osteoarthritis, fibromyalgia, rheumatoid arthritis and gout. The knowledge that four distinct conditions are responsible for the majority of rheumatic type pain is not often understood today, let alone hundreds of years ago. It is now known that fibromyalgia is the second most common rheumatologic disorder behind osteoarthritis.[2]

In the past, it was believed that all rheumatic type pains were variations of gout. Even though this is not actually true, doctors, healers and herbalists were extremely perceptive and by the 1700s had found four treatments that were effective at treating these four causes of rheumatism. It is only now in hindsight that we can see that each of these four treatments specifically correlates with one of the four causes of rheumatic-type pains.

A rheumatology book, *The Textbook of the Rheumatic Diseases*, discusses these four most widely used treatments for rheumatic pain in the 1700s. The treatments listed are sulfur, guaiac (the herbal forerunner of guaifenesin), colchicum, and quinine.[3] Although other medical treatments of this era were ineffective and dangerous—such as bleeding and mercury—the therapeutic values of these four approaches is still recognized. In fact, these four treatments that were preferred hundreds of years ago still serve as the foundation for many of our current medications in the treatment of osteoarthritis, fibromyalgia, rheumatoid arthritis and gout. These treatments were so far ahead of their time that the therapeutic benefits of sulfur and guaiac were lost for hundreds of years (due to in large part to the complexities of diagnosis that are associated with rheumatic conditions and continue to be a stumbling block even to this day) and not rediscovered until after 1980. Here is a review of these medications and the conditions that they help.

- Quinine is well known as a treatment for malaria, but it was also used to treat rheumatoid arthritis.[4] It has given rise to new quinine-like drug, hydroxychloroquine, also known as plaquenil. This is one of the few drugs useful in the long-term treatment of rheumatoid arthritis.
- Colchicum, or meadow saffron, used in Hippocrate's time for gout and written of extensively, was forgotten or ignored for

unknown reasons for over 2000 years. It is now used to obtain colchicine, a medicine still used today for treatment of the symptoms of acute gout.[5]

- Sulfur in the form of glucosamine sulfate, chondroitin sulfate, and methylsulfonylmethane (MSM) was rediscovered in the 1980s as being helpful for osteoarthritis. These products are now safely helping thousands of people.[6] Although these forms of sulfur are relatively new, one could argue that the use of sulfur for treating osteoarthritis has been rediscovered.

- Guaiac from the guaiacum tree is repeatedly mentioned as a treatment for rheumatism in historical medical texts.[7,8] It is now available as guaifenesin, and is helping many people with fibromyalgia and related nonplus conditions. Like sulfur, after the 1800s guaiac was largely forgotten.

The history of rheumatism has consisted of teasing out the individual conditions responsible for causing rheumatic type pains that involve the joints and surrounding tissues. The first condition that was identified as a cause for rheumatism, by Hippocrates, was gout. As previously mentioned, until the mid 1900s physicians were rarely able to distinguish different types of rheumatism and until the late 1800s considered them all to be variants of gout.[9] Over two thousand years passed from the time of Hippocrates before two more conditions—rheumatoid arthritis and osteoarthritis—were recognized as being separate from gout and achieved wide recognition in health care. Fibromyalgia is the last primary cause of rheumatism to be recognized. Because fibromyalgia lacks some of the more obvious characteristic features that are present in gout, rheumatoid arthritis and osteoarthritis, many physicians even to this day refuse to acknowledge its existence. Over the centuries, only a few doctors have been able to recognize fibromyalgia as a separate entity and suggest a name. A few of the names that have been used for what we now call fibromyalgia are fibrositis, myofibrositis, nonarticular rheumatism, and myositis. The matter of what to call fibromyalgia and how to classify this type of pain and malfunction with its myriad symptoms persists even to this day.[10]

Using guaifenesin to treat fibromyalgia and the other nonplus conditions may seem strange to some people, especially physicians. This is because in modern times guaifenesin is known only as an expectorant. Because of these expectorant qualities, it is contained in most cough syrups. This has lead to ridicule of guaifenesin when used to treat the nonplus conditions as the "cough syrup cure," with the implication that nothing could be more ridiculous. Yet, for anyone who has had the symptoms of the nonplus conditions relieved by guaifenesin, there can be no doubt that it is effective. It also appears clear that the reason guaiac was used as a treatment for rheumatism centuries ago is because it was treating fibromyalgia. With the recovery of ancient knowledge, we can see that fibromyalgia is not a modern disease, but is as old as gout and arthritis.

For centuries, until the guaiacum tree became rare from overcutting, guaiac (sometimes referred to as guaiacum or guiacol) was derived from the sap or resin of this tree.[11,12] The knowledge that guaiac was helpful for some types of rheumatic pains and for sore throats because it loosens thick phlegm has been around since the mid 1500s.[13] In modern times guaifenesin has only been recognized as an expectorant since the 1970s. Guaifenesin's ability to treat fibromyalgia has been obscured, in part because fibromyalgia as a health problem has remained misunderstood and unrecognized, but also because the use of salicylate containing compounds in soap, tooth paste and other commonly used products is much more common today than in the 1500s. Salicylate containing products can block guaifenesin's effectiveness.

The story of fibromyalgia and guaiac and now fibromyalgia and guaifenesin has, in a way reversed itself over the centuries. From the 1500s to the 1800s, guaiac was used as a treatment for aches and pains that had no particular name except the catchall term rheumatism. Now we have the improved understanding that allows us to identify and name the individual causes for rheumatic type pains, but an effective treatment used centuries ago remains unrecognized. Thus we have the irony that some of the most confusing disorders of modern times, fibromyalgia, and the other nonplus conditions, were treated more effectively 300 years ago than they are today.

It was not until 1992 that Paul St. Amand, M.D., rediscovered guaiac's therapeutic benefits through guaifenesin.[14] These benefits were possible because he recognized that when treating fibromyalgia, guaifenesin might be salicylate sensitive, (like some gout medications), and that guaifenesin should be dosed gradually and carefully. He also learned that reactive hypoglycemia is a common co-condition of the nonplus conditions and should be addressed when present. Results using guaifenesin are not likely unless one adjusts to these three factors.

In the 1820s willow and other herbs that contained salicylates in significant amounts began to be used more extensively.[15] Salicylates, the forerunner of aspirin are unique in that they are able to often provide relief, even if only temporary, for all of the primary rheumatic conditions (gout, rheumatoid arthritis, fibromyalgia and osteoarthritis). The effectiveness of salicylates likely overshadowed the other common treatments of the day particularly sulfur and guaiac. This is especially true since salicylates could reduce the symptoms of all four of the common causes of rheumatism while the other treatments previously discussed had to be paired with the correct condition if it was to be of any benefit. Pairing one of the four rheumatic conditions with the correct treatment is unlikely since the ability to consistently differentiate between the rheumatic conditions was not possible. This made salicylates appear to be more effective, or at least more consistent as a treatment. In addition, since salicylates block the effectiveness of guaifenesin and presumably guaiac as well, anyone using salicylate would no longer find guaiac helpful. Acetylsalicylic acid (aspirin) was discovered in 1897, largely replacing natural sources of salicylate and ushered in the modern pharmaceutical era.

Aspirin, and salicylates in general, have a complex and unique relationship to gout, osteoarthritis, rheumatoid arthritis, and fibromyalgia. First, salicylates from natural sources, and later aspirin, were among the first medications that consistently and significantly relieved muscle and joint pain, whether from rheumatic conditions or from soft tissue injury and joint misalignment. In addition, aspirin and other salicylates impact gout and fibromyalgia in several other unique ways. It is well known that low levels of salicylates can decrease uric acid excretion and cause gout in susceptible individuals. Another confusing aspect is that there is a variable response to salicylate usage for people with gout and fibromyalgia with the result being that salicylates can provide temporary relief as well as cause an aggravation of symptoms in both conditions.

If that wasn't confusing enough, high levels of aspirin can actually help the kidneys to excrete uric acid although this is not considered a safe way to treat gout because of side effects associated with aspirin. Another surprise is that guaifenesin is able to mildly increase the excretion of uric acid and is known as a mild uricosuric agent.[16] This effect of guaifenesin on uric acid is so small that it is not used as a treatment for gout. Stronger uricosuric medications exist that help the kidneys to excrete uric acid in meaningful amounts, but these medications are also rendered ineffective by aspirin use. With all of the similarities between gout and fibromyalgia and the medications that treat these conditions, it should come as no surprise that salicylates can also block guaifenesin's therapeutic effects when treating fibromyalgia and the nonplus conditions.

Incidentally, guaifenesin's mucus-thinning properties are not affected by salicylates. When used to treat nonplus conditions, however, guaifenesin is extremely sensitive to even lower levels of salicylates than are the uricosuric medications used to treat gout. During the years of using guaifenesin in my practice, I have had dozens of patients with one or more of the nonplus conditions who have found that once all sources of salicylates are eliminated, significant improvement takes place even before guaifenesin is started. How to avoid salicylates is covered in detail in Chapter 7. It is likely that guaifenesin's sensitivity to very low levels of salicylates has contributed to keeping the benefits of guaifenesin hidden. This explains why no doctor or researcher has inadvertently rediscovered guaifenesin to be helpful, in spite of the fact that guaifenesin use in the general population has been common since the 1970s.

My experience of repeatedly seeing guaifenesin eliminate symptoms caused not only by fibromyalgia, but also by all of the nonplus conditions, has helped me to recognize how closely these conditions are related. In the next chapter I explore the four basic traits shared by the nonplus conditions.

4

Nonplus Conditions: Different symptoms; one cause

Much is known about the individual nonplus conditions, yet an understanding of how these different conditions are related is not widely grasped. Based on the names and symptoms of the nonplus conditions it is not obvious that they share many important traits. Recognizing the interrelationships between these conditions can be a revelation to a person who is experiencing many different health problems. When it is discovered that a great many of their symptoms are actually the result of one underlying problem, people often feel less baffled by their health problems. It can also be helpful to physicians who have been overwhelmed by the number and variety of symptoms in their patients who have several of the nonplus conditions.

When I found out that the burning pain between my shoulders was related to exhaustion after exercise, which in turn was related to my occasional off-balance days, difficulty sleeping, that fiendish itching of my forearms at night, and my chemical sensitivities, my life suddenly made much more sense. For some reason I felt comfort in knowing I did not have 20 different problems, but one problem with twenty different manifestations. Most of my symptoms began at different times of my life. Each symptom had a different intensity and frequency of occurrence. It certainly did not seem that they were connected. In fact, I was not convinced that this was actually true until I personally experienced the changes that took place in all of these symptoms after taking guaifenesin.

In this chapter I show why these 10 conditions can be grouped together and why it is likely that they have the same underlying cause. All of the nonplus conditions are listed here alphabetically with the common name first. After the commonly used name, I have also included a few of the better known and sometimes inaccurate synonyms.

Chronic Fatigue Syndrome (CFS), Chronic Fatigue and Immune Dysfunction Syndrome (CFIDS), Candidiasis, Chronic Epstein-Barr Virus (EBV), Myalgic Encephalitis (ME), Myalgic Encephalomyelitis, Yuppie Flu, Neurasthenia

Ehlers-Danlos Syndrome (EDS), Loose Joints, Loose Ligaments

Fibromyalgia Syndrome (FMS), Fibrositis, Fibromyositis, Myositis, Nonarticular Rheumatism

Interstitial Cystitis (IC), Irritable Bladder, Pelvic Pain Syndrome,

Irritable Bowel Syndrome (IBS), Sensitive Bowel, Functional Bowel Disease

Multiple Chemical Sensitivity (MCS), Chemically Sensitive, Chemical Sensitivities, Environmental Illness (EI)

Neurally Mediated Hypotension (NMH), Orthostatic Intolerance (OI), Postural Hypotension

Restless Leg Syndrome (RLS), Periodic Limb Movement Disorder (PLMD)

Vulvodynia (VV), Vulvar Pain Syndrome, Pelvic Pain Syndrome

The four traits common to all of these conditions are:

1. Shared symptoms and overlapping of conditions.
2. Method of diagnosis.
3. Treatment difficulty.
4. Guaifenesin as an effective treatment.

1. Shared symptoms.

It is possible for an individual to have only one nonplus condition that results in just one symptom. It is much more common for a person to have more than one nonplus condition resulting in several symptoms and often several dozen symptoms. This is especially true for people who are unlucky enough to have three or four or more of the nonplus conditions.

It is helpful to think of three of the nonplus conditions as being core conditions: chronic fatigue/chronic fatigue and immune dysfunction, fibromyalgia, and irritable bowel. This is because they are the most common and are more likely to occur alone without the symptoms of the other nonplus conditions. The remaining nonplus conditions can be considered satellite conditions. The satellite conditions may occur alone, but commonly attend one or all three of the core nonplus conditions.

If you have one of the core conditions then you are likely to also have one or more of the satellite nonplus conditions. Many books, websites, and research articles that discuss one of the nonplus conditions comment on how they frequently occur with other conditions. In most cases, the conditions that are mentioned are nonplus conditions. Some authorities suggest a common underlying mechanism is responsible for all of these conditions.[1,2,3,4,5]

Not only do the nonplus conditions frequently occur together, but their symptoms frequently overlap as well. For example, difficulty sleeping, muscle aches, and problems with memory and thinking are frequent in chronic fatigue, fibromyalgia, restless legs and multiple chemical sensitivities.

2. Similar method of diagnosis.

Diagnosing nearly all of the nonplus conditions is difficult for two reasons. First, many symptoms that are common in the nonplus conditions are also present in dozens of other disorders. Back pain and fatigue are two symptoms that have many possible causes. Second, at this time no diagnostic technology such as x-ray, ultrasound, MRI, electroencephalogram or laboratory test can identify the nonplus conditions. The diagnosis for all nonplus conditions is based primarily upon an inability to find a reason for their existence, as well as an inability to find an effective treatment.

The negative tests do serve to rule out other disorders that could be responsible for the same symptoms. As I previously mentioned, this ruling out process may take many years. It is not uncommon for a person to see dozens of doctors from many different specialties over a period of four or five or even ten years before a nonplus condition is accurately diagnosed.

Some of the nonplus conditions are not difficult to diagnose due to a symptom that is particularly unique. For example, restless legs syndrome is easily identified since its only symptom is an uncontrollable urge to move the legs. In addition, the diagnosis of this condition is made easier by the fact that there are few other conditions that cause this.

One of the nonplus conditions, Ehlers-Danlos Syndrome, does have a known cause in a small percent of all cases. Ten percent of Ehlers-Danlos Syndrome cases are due to an identifiable genetic defect.[6] I do not recommend guaifenesin in these cases.

It can be claimed that one of the nonplus conditions, neurally mediated hypotension, has a specific test that can identify it. While it is true that the tilt table test will be positive when this condition is present, this test merely confirms the symptoms already described by the patient. It does little to shed light on what is causing this symptom. Even when the test is positive, the diagnosis is still based upon the symptoms experienced by the patient. Another weakness of the test is that it is only likely to detect neurally mediated hypotension when the patient is actively experiencing the symptoms. Like many of the nonplus conditions, neurally mediated hypotension may be experienced on an intermittent basis. This makes it possible for the test to be negative when in reality the condition is present, but not active at the time of the test. When a test fails to identify a condition that is actually present, it is called a false negative.

The primary benefit of the tilt table test is that it may objectively confirm the reality of the patient's subjective complaint. It is unfortunate that more tests are not available that can objectively confirm other symptoms like fatigue, pain, and digestive distress. If this were possible then sufferers of these conditions would be treated with greater consideration.

The American College of Rheumatology has established criteria for fibromyalgia diagnosis that includes both a history of chronic widespread pain in all four quadrants of the body and the presence of nine of 18 "tender points" on physical examination. This test is widely known and used, but it is not generally known that "These criteria were never intended to be strictly applied to individual patients as diagnostic criteria, and it is widely acknowledged that many persons who have the clinical diagnosis of fibromyalgia do not fulfill this definition."[7] When physicians do strictly apply these criteria the result is a significant number of false negatives meaning that some patients who actually have fibromyalgia will show up negative based on these criteria, and thus are inaccurately told that they do not have fibromyalgia.

I, for one, failed to have pain in all four quadrants, nor did I have nine out of 18 "tender points" present. An alternative to the eighteen tender points is a procedure called mapping. Mapping, a term used by Paul St. Amand, M.D. acknowledges the historical and modern findings that fibromyalgia is often associated with a bumpy feeling under the skin that is often tender as well.[8] It was William Balfour, M.D. of Edinburgh who in 1816 first mentioned the occurrence of "indurated nodules" associated with "rheumatism."[9]

It is now recognized by most doctors using guaifenesin that these lumps and bumps occur not only with fibromyalgia but are present in all of the nonplus conditions. Mapping is the process of running fingers down the muscles of the body and charting where the lumps and bumps are located. The bumps can feel like small pebbles or larger hardened areas and swellings. The bumps may be easily felt and are often sensitive, but can require an experienced doctor or therapist to be found. It should be noted that the number and size of these swellings does not seem to be directly related to the severity of the symptoms one experiences.

These lumps and bumps do not include lymph nodes, lipomas, cellulite, or tight muscles. Mapping should not be used as a sole means of diagnosis for any of the nonplus conditions.

3. Treatments have limited benefit.

Many of the symptoms resulting from nonplus conditions are not unusual. Fatigue, headaches, muscle aches, and pains are almost universal, and there are many helpful treatments available depending upon the source of the problem. Exercise, relaxation, soft tissue therapy, adjustments, vitamins, and medications can control or eliminate these symptoms in most instances. However, when these symptoms and others are due to any of the nonplus conditions, not only is there no detectable reason for the pain, but common treatments provide little if any long-term relief, and the overall progression of various aches, pains, fatigue, and digestive upset continues. Even if one symptom is alleviated due to a specific treatment, or disappears for no reason at all, the other symptoms remain and new symptoms may arrive at any time.

4. Guaifenesin eliminates the symptoms associated with the nonplus conditions.

When guaifenesin is used with three specific therapeutic steps, the symptoms of these conditions gradually decrease over time and are often eliminated completely. This is a gradual process and while most people will experience significant improvement within several weeks to several months, complete recovery will take many years in most cases. Although no treatment or therapy is 100 percent effective in all cases, it has been my experience that guaifenesin helps the vast majority of people who use it properly. It is safe, inexpensive, and in most instances can gradually eliminate all of the symptoms resulting from the nonplus conditions.

Unfortunately, most doctors who try guaifenesin on their patients simply prescribe 2400 milligrams of guaifenesin daily—the amount commonly used for expectorant purposes—and know nothing about the required therapeutic steps of proper dosing, salicylate avoidance, and carbohydrate sensitivity. Symptom improvement under these circumstances is highly unlikely.

The existence of these four important traits shows that the nonplus conditions are closely connected. Most of these conditions have other similarities as well. The majority of the nonplus conditions affect women at a significantly higher rate and are believed to have a genetic component.

In the next chapter, I discuss one theory that was developed to explain the cause of the nonplus conditions, and how guaifenesin works to reverse them.

5

Phosphate Retention Theory

There are many theories about the causes of the various nonplus conditions. These theories blame everything from alterations of brain chemistry to sleep disorders to trigger points. No theory has been proven or even widely accepted. One theory however is unique, because it explains how a particular chemical imbalance could cause any of the nonplus conditions. It also provides an explanation of how guaifenesin works and why it is salicylate sensitive.

The phosphate retention theory has been proposed by Paul St. Amand, M.D. to explain the cause of fibromyalgia and many of the nonplus conditions as well as why guaifenesin is therapeutic for them.[1] This is the same doctor who rediscovered guaifenesin as an effective treatment for fibromyalgia. He believes that the symptoms of these conditions are due to a gradual accumulation of excess phosphate in the cells of the body due to a malfunction in the kidneys.

The mineral phosphorus does not exist in a pure state in nature, but is found in combination with calcium to form phosphate. Phosphate is an essential mineral in the human body, but like anything else, too much causes problems. A primary point of this theory is that excess phosphates disrupt normal cell and organ function, eventually creating malfunction and symptoms. If a person does not eliminate phosphate normally through excretion via the kidneys, it can slowly accumulate. As time goes on, more and more cells throughout the body are forced to store the excess phosphate. This creates an expanding array of symptoms wherever the excess phosphates are being stored. For example, mental fogginess, sleep disorders, and depression associated with fibromyalgia, chronic fatigue and multiple chemical sensitivity would indicate that excess phosphate is being stored in the brain. Irritable bowel symptoms could be due to phosphate storage in the digestive tract and so on.

Excess phosphate storage not only creates symptoms throughout the body, but also is thought to be responsible for the lumps and bumps found on people with the nonplus conditions. The cells storing the excess phosphate respond by retaining water, causing the lumps and bumps. The cause of this phosphate retention is believed to be the result of an inherited inability of the kidneys to excrete phosphate normally. Although the kidneys are still excreting some phosphate, they are doing so at a slightly less than optimum rate. This forces the cells in the body to gradually store phosphate. Blood tests will not show high levels of phosphate because the body does not store excess phosphate in the blood. According to this theory, guaifenesin is beneficial because it binds to receptor sites within the kidneys resulting in an increased rate of phosphate excretion. As the kidneys, with the help of guaifenesin, eliminate more phosphate, the cells in the body that have been storing excess phosphate can begin to release it. Because guaifenesin does not repair the kidneys themselves, it is not a cure and must be continually taken to maintain proper phosphate elimination.

Guaifenesin does not work well when salicylates are in the body. This is because the receptor sites in the kidney, where the molecules of guaifenesin attach, bind with salicylates more easily than with guaifenesin. Thus, when salicylates are present they occupy the receptor sites, preventing guaifenesin from reaching its destination and having its desired effect. This results in salicylates partially blocking or completely blocking guaifenesin.

It is also postulated that the cause of symptoms is not just from the storage of excess phosphate in the cells, but is also from the movement of excess phosphate into and out of the cells. This may explain why one particular symptom such as low back pain may be persistent for years, while the body stores phosphates in this area. Then, when phosphate storage shifts to a new location, symptoms in the low back may diminish while a different set of symptoms develop at the new storage site.

Movement of phosphate out of the cells as a result of guaifenesin's effect on the kidneys can recreate the same pain that was present during the storage of phosphates in a particular area. This accounts for the temporary exacerbations of current symptoms as well as the temporary return of symptoms that may not have been experienced in years when guaifenesin is used.

Thus the phosphate retention theory explains:

1. What causes fibromyalgia as well as all of the nonplus conditions.
2. Why such a wide variety of conditions and symptoms could take place as a result of one underlying malfunction.
3. Why symptoms of these conditions may be intermittent or disappear completely and sometimes seem to be replaced by new symptoms.
4. Why guaifenesin could be therapeutic and yet at the same time cause a temporary increase in some symptoms.
5. What is the cause of the lumps and bumps that can usually be found on the surface of the bodies of people who have these conditions.
6. Why guaifenesin is blocked by salicylates.

A temporary increase of symptoms brought on by appropriate treatment is not unique in medicine. A similar situation occurs in the medical condition known as gout. In fact there are many similarities between gout and the nonplus conditions some of which were covered in chapter 3. Reviewing these similarities shows that gout serves as precedent for many of the ideas in the phosphate retention theory. This is all the more interesting since both gout and fibromyalgia are conditions that historically fall under the banner of chronic rheumatism.[2]

A comparison of gout and the nonplus conditions proves interesting. Gout is due to an excess of uric acid in the body, while nonplus conditions may be due to excess phosphates. Gout symptoms increase as excess uric acid accumulates in various tissues over time, and symptoms increase in the various locations in the body where the uric acid crystals accumulate. In the nonplus conditions, symptoms increase as phosphates are stored in various body locations and create symptoms in these areas. Drugs that treat gout by helping the kidneys to increase the excretion of uric acid frequently set off an increase in gout symptoms. This is similar to how taking guaifenesin can create a temporary increase in symptoms as it stimulates the kidneys to excrete phosphates. Gout medication must be used in such a way as to effectively lower uric acid, but must be done gradually enough to avoid excessively increasing symptoms. Guaifenesin also is dosed slowly and gradually so as to not unnecessarily increase symptoms. The drugs that treat gout by lowering uric acid levels are blocked by salicylates. Guaifenesin is also blocked by salicylates, and is even sensitive to very low levels of salicylates. Lastly, the symptoms of gout can be aggravated and even caused by the use of aspirin or other salicylates. Similarly, there are some people with nonplus conditions who feel improvement simply by eliminating salicylates and become worse when salicylate exposure is increased.

The phosphate retention theory has not been proven and may not be completely accurate. However, it does provide an explanation of why and how guaifenesin works. If part or even all of the phosphate retention theory is disproven at some point in the future, it does not change the fact that guaifenesin is a significant help for most people who use it correctly. It should be remembered that there are many effective medications used in health care even though little or nothing is known as to why they work.

I have read several articles by people who believe that they have disproven the phosphate retention theory and dismiss guaifenesin as an effective therapy. It should be remembered that the phosphate retention theory is an attempt to explain *how* guaifenesin is therapeutic, not *if* it is therapeutic. There is no denying that guaifenesin has worked for thousands of people worldwide. In my own practice I have seen hundreds of people recover from the nonplus conditions. Often, these were patients that had seen many doctors for a period of 10 or even 20 years. In spite of dozens of therapies and treatments, guaifenesin and guaifenesin alone was able to create long-term improvement of all symptoms.

6

What to expect when taking guaifenesin and how to get started

A common misconception regarding guaifenesin is that it is necessary to feel much worse before symptom improvement occurs. After starting more than 600 patients on guaifenesin, I have seen that the most common initial response is for some symptoms to improve while others worsen. If the dose is correct, any increase in symptoms is unlikely to be greater than what has been experienced in the past. As time goes on and guaifenesin use is continued, more and more symptoms improve or are eliminated. If on the other hand, the guaifenesin dose is excessive, an unnecessary increase in the pains and other symptoms associated with the nonplus conditions is likely to take place. In the vast majority of people, when guaifenesin is dosed properly, there is no need to feel much worse month after month in order to experience long lasting improvement.

I have found that most people taking guaifenesin for the nonplus conditions will experience significant improvements of at least one symptom and often several symptoms within one to six weeks after the proper dose has been found. It is important to be aware that using guaifenesin requires considerable participation by the person using it in order for the required steps to be followed successfully. If you are looking for a quick fix that requires nothing more than swallowing a pill, then guaifenesin may not be for you.

If, however, you are willing to take an active role in your recovery, then it is likely that guaifenesin will work for you. How a person experiences recovery using guaifenesin varies almost as much as the symptoms of the nonplus conditions. Some lucky people feel a rapid improvement of every symptom while most people respond by a slow and gradual improvement of symptoms interspersed by temporary increases of some of their symptoms. There are also people whose initial symptom changes involve only an aggravation of one or more symptoms for weeks before some improvement is felt. Even in these instances, significant improvement of at least one symptom usually takes place within six weeks.

Another way of feeling improvement is in terms of good hours, days, or weeks. A good week is where several symptoms, or even all symptoms, are much improved. As guaifenesin continues to be taken, the good days become more common. Regardless of what type of initial response you experience, it is likely that some symptoms will take several months or years before responding to guaifenesin. How long it takes a specific symptom to respond to guaifenesin may depend upon how long that symptom has been present. In some, but not all instances, symptoms that have been present for many years take longer to respond. It is not known why 10 to 20 percent of people using guaifenesin for the nonplus conditions may not respond at all.

It should be clear by now that taking guaifenesin does not suddenly make the nonplus conditions disappear. According to the phosphate retention theory, taking guaifenesin stops the accumulation of phosphates by acting on the kidneys in a way that helps the body to increase the amount of phosphate that is eliminated. Stopping the accumulation of phosphate is important, but the time consuming aspect of using guaifenesin lies in eliminating all of the phosphate that has been stored in the body over a persons lifetime. This phosphate elimination process takes many years depending upon age. In general, the older a person is the more phosphate they have accumulated, thus the longer it takes to eliminate the phosphate load.

The nonplus conditions are believed to be genetic. When people are born with the inability to excrete phosphate normally, every year of life more phosphate is stored. The age at which a person begins to express symptoms is dependent upon the rate at which phosphate is being stored and where it is being stored. Although it is common for a person to blame an injury or illness for starting one of the nonplus conditions, it is believed that nonplus symptoms would have begun even without the traumatic event or illness in these people.

As a result of improved kidney function from guaifenesin, it is theorized that every month of taking guaifenesin eliminates approximately seven months of phosphate storage. Likewise, every year of guaifenesin use eliminates about seven years worth of phosphates. Of course this is just a rough estimate since some people, presumably those with more severe cases, have been storing phosphate more rapidly and will take longer to deplete their phosphate stores. People with less severe cases likely store phosphate more slowly, so they will eliminate their stored phosphate more rapidly. Because all of the excess phosphates are not immediately eliminated by guaifenesin, neither are all of the symptoms. Taking guaifenesin can be compared to playing a tape of a movie in reverse. As guaifenesin decreases the level of stored phosphates it is like turning back the clock, except the clock reverses seven times more quickly.

For example, as a result of taking guaifenesin for one month, symptoms will reverse to where they were approximately seven months ago. In the same vein, symptoms that were prominent 14 years ago may once again resurface after being on guaifenesin for two years. Not all symptoms backtrack through time in this way, and some people never experience this type of temporary resurgence of symptoms, but instead feel changes in some of the ways already described above.

Because the nonplus conditions usually cause a wide variety of different symptoms, it can be hard to remember how different symptoms are changing as a result of taking guaifenesin. It is especially easy to forget symptoms that have lessened or are gone completely since they are no longer reminding you of their presence. Making a record of all your symptoms that are associated with the nonplus conditions before you start taking guaifenesin can help you to recognize when and how much improvement has taken place.

There is a symptom summary provided on page ix at the beginning of the book. If you are already using guaifenesin, use the symptom summary to record the status of what your symptoms were before you started taking guaifenesin. Referring to this sheet frequently, especially when first taking guaifenesin, should make it easier to recognize at what dose your symptoms start changing. This is the signal that you are at or near your proper dose of guaifenesin.

Remember, it is normal if you find some symptoms are aggravated by guaifenesin for periods of time, and it is possible that a few symptoms will remain unchanged for months and possibly years. If this happens, try to focus on the symptoms that have improved or have been completely eliminated. With time and continued use, the vast majority of people find that more and more symptoms begin to moderate with either decreasing frequency or intensity.

Guaifenesin as a treatment for the nonplus conditions is far from perfect, just like many other treatments that are used for health conditions from cancer to arthritis. Treatments for these and other common diseases may involve drugs that are helpful yet toxic, and surgery that is risky, yet unavoidable. When compared to these conditions and their standard medical treatments, using guaifenesin to treat the nonplus conditions is very safe and relatively simple. Actually, there are many ways that guaifenesin is an ideal treatment. It is an inexpensive and safe medication. It is neither habit-forming nor does the dose need to be raised over time to remain effective. As a nonprescription medication it does not usually require doctor supervision, although a knowledgeable doctor can help ensure success.

Guaifenesin does not appear to be a cure. It helps the body in some way, possibly by increasing the elimination of phosphates, but it does not restore proper function permanently. Some individuals who use guaifenesin get such rapid and complete relief that after a year or two all symptoms have been eliminated. In such instances these patients may want to stop guaifenesin or may just forget to take it regularly, since they no longer have consistent symptoms. In almost all instances, these people find that their symptoms return after they have discontinued guaifenesin for a period of time. Maintaining one's therapeutic dose appears to be the only way to prevent symptoms from recurring.

Guaifenesin is a commonly used medication and most people have taken it occasionally, even if they did not know it. This is because guaifenesin is contained in most cold and flu remedies. Guaifenesin is best known as an expectorant. Expectorants help to loosen mucus (phlegm) and thin bronchial secretions. This helps the bronchial tubes to drain and makes coughs more productive. Many doctors will also recommend guaifenesin to help drain congested sinuses. When people find it to be helpful for sinus problems, it may be taken daily for decades. Guaifenesin is well tolerated and has a wide margin of safety. Side effects have been generally mild and infrequent, especially when compared to other medications or even to some vitamins and herbs.

There are several differences between taking guaifenesin for mucus thinning and using it to treat the nonplus conditions. First, mucus thinning generally requires higher doses of guaifenesin. The dose recommendations written on bottles of guaifenesin are for use as an expectorant. When using guaifenesin to treat nonplus conditions, considerably less guaifenesin is usually needed for optimum results. Second, drinking extra water while taking guaifenesin is a step a person can take that may help thin mucus, but is not necessary when treating the nonplus conditions. Instead, different steps are essential.

The three steps to using guaifenesin are:

1. Acquiring an understanding of what salicylates are, as well as how to avoid salicylates both internally and externally.
2. Understanding how to find one's therapeutic dose of guaifenesin. The recommended dose on the bottle is for expectorant purposes and is frequently higher than necessary for the treatment of nonplus conditions.
3. Knowing how to treat reactive hypoglycemia with the necessry diet changes if certain symptoms are experienced after eating sugary and starchy foods. Sleepiness, brain fog, anxiety, irritability, insomnia, cravings for sweets or snacks, bloating, gas, and other digestive problems are some of the common symptoms associated with reactive hypoglycemia. Reactive hypoglycemia is present in approximately 40 percent of the women and 20

percent of the men with a nonplus condition. The symptoms of reactive hypoglycemia mimic many of the same symptoms caused by the nonplus conditions. When these symptoms flair up due to excessive carbohydrate consumption, it can create confusion about whether or not guaifenesin is working. Decreasing sugars and starches in your diet is recommended if you experience reactive hypoglycemia, sometimes referred to as carbohydrate sensitivity.

In most cases, your doctor will not be familiar with these three steps, nor will there be an understanding of why they are necessary when using guaifenesin to treat the nonplus conditions. I have had many people tell me that the doctor who recommended they give guaifenesin a try did not discuss salicylates, dosing, or reactive hypoglycemia. In these cases it is likely that the doctor is simply passing on information heard from colleagues or patients. Because many doctors are familiar with guaifenesin as an expectorant and know it is safe, they may recommend it without knowing anything about how to use it effectively. As well meaning as these doctors are, their actions are creating legions of patients who now believe that guaifenesin is of no help, simply because they did not know how to use it properly.

Because most doctors have no knowledge of these important steps, it is up to you to learn how to effectively use guaifenesin. Only a lucky few will find a physician who is truly knowledgeable and experienced in this area, and even in these cases you still need to know this information for yourself.

7

The salicylate problem or step one: avoiding salicylates

Salicylates (sah-LISS-a-lates) are a common but relatively unknown type of chemical that the average person is exposed to on a daily basis. If a person is familiar with the term they are likely to think of aspirin, yet there are other more common—if less potent—sources of exposure to salicylates from toothpaste to sunscreen. There are many types of salicylates; some are manufactured and some are from natural plant sources. All the different types of salicylates must be avoided for guaifenesin to be effective. Plants produce varying amounts of salicylates as a way of defending themselves from soil bacteria.[1] Salicylates are also manufactured synthetically for use in a wide variety of products from shampoo to pain relievers. When salicylates enter the blood stream, whether from a natural or man-made source, they have the ability to stop or block guaifenesin's therapeutic benefits for the nonplus conditions. This blocking can occur anytime salicylate exposure occurs. Once in the system, salicylates continue to block for approximately 24 hours.

Because avoiding salicylates requires discontinuing some brands of products commonly used, from vitamins to mouthwash, people may be inclined to skip this step. This is not a good idea. One of the most common reasons for poor results or sporadic success using guaifenesin is that salicylates were not eliminated or only avoided in a halfhearted way.

When persons learn about guaifenesin they are often motivated to start using it immediately. I understand the sense of urgency, but it is best to take the time to learn about and eliminate salicylates before taking guaifenesin. Tens of thousands of people have used guaifenesin over the years as an expectorant and there is no doubt that a percentage of them had one or more of the nonplus conditions. The primary reason that guaifenesin was not noticed as being helpful for the nonplus conditions is because exposure to salicylates through products used by people everyday is universal. It appears that Dr. St. Amand is the first physician in modern times to recognize the benefits of guaifenesin, in part because he understood that it was salicylate sensitive.[2]

Salicylates enter the body in two ways: by mouth and through the skin via lotions, soap, or other products placed on the skin, gums, and scalp. Surprisingly, salicylates enter the blood stream through the skin more easily than they do when eaten. This is because when a substance is swallowed the liver eliminates low levels of salicylates, such as found in food (fruit and vegetables). Greater amounts of salicylates such as is found in aspirin, also known as acetylsalicylic acid, medicinal herbs, in the form of either pills or tea and breath sprays or breath mints (all types of mints are especially strong in salicylates) will not immediately be eliminated by the liver. When the liver cannot eliminate all of the salicylates then some of the salicylates will enter the blood stream and guaifenesin will be blocked. There is frequently confusion regarding food so I will repeat—all foods can be eaten without posing a problem with regard to salicylates, and even spices can be used in normal amounts as a part of food preparation.

Many products that we put on our skin contains enough salicylates to block guaifenesin. Salicylates that enter through the skin or gums do not pass through through the liver before entering the blood. This is why it is acceptable to eat fruit and vegetables, but when using a product that is placed on the body it must not contains any type of plant extract. Salicylates from both natural (plant) and synthetic sources will readily penetrate our skin, scalp, lips, or gums, and from there enter the bloodstream much more readily than when eaten. It is well known that salicylates pass through the skin, which is one reason why topical pain relievers are often effective. For example, the active ingredient in Aspercreme is trolamine salicylate.

The scope of the problem becomes apparent when we realize that many of the products we place on our skin or gums contain a wide range of botanicals such as herb, fruit, and plant extracts. With few exceptions, any ingredient derived from plant sources will likely contain enough salicylates to block guaifenesin if applied to the body. Most toothpaste, sunscreen, makeup, and other toiletries, when placed on the skin are likely to block unless you are careful to choose the appropriate products.

Synthetic salicylates may also be contained in these products and penetrate the skin just as easily. Octyl-salicylate, for example, the active ingredient in most sunscreens, is a synthetic salicylate and a potent blocker. This particular chemical is easy to recognize as a salicylate because the word "salicylate" is part of its name. Unfortunately, many synthetic salicylates do not have the word salicylate contained in their name. Some examples are orthohydroxybenzoate and o-carboxyphenol. By learning how to find and use salicylate-free products you can eliminate salicylate exposure and greatly increase your chances of success. If you are concerned about learning complex terms, don't worry, you will not need to memorize dozens of chemical names. Finding salicylate-free products has been made easy and is discussed below.

Once salicylate molecules are in the bloodstream, they will soon come into contact with special receptor sites in the kidneys. The salicylate molecules, according to the phosphate retention theory, have a high affinity for the same receptor sites in the kidneys that are needed for guaifenesin to work. This enables salicylates to push the guaifenesin aside, rendering it ineffective.

To review, there are two major ways in which contact with salicylates can become a problem:

1. *Entering through the skin.* Unless you carefully choose salicylate-free products this can occur with most anything that you put on your skin, scalp, lips, gums, or hold inside of your mouth.

Substances may include soaps, sunscreens, cosmetics, toothpaste, flavored dental floss, baby wipes, and even chewing tobacco. If you are using a medication that is put on the skin, check all ingredients for salicylates. Gardening/weeding with bare hands is also a problem since plants contain salicylates on their exterior surface. Wear gloves, or if gardening for only a short period of time wash your hands afterwards.

2. *Entering by ingestion.* Aspirin or products containing aspirin will block guaifenesin. Herbal supplements and most teas that claim to have medicinal value have a high enough concentration of salicylates to block. Vitamins that contain herbs should also be discontinued. However, coffee, black tea and green tea are usually low enough in salicylates for most people to use, although people who are very salicylate sensitive may need to avoid these as well. All foods, as well as herbs, when used as seasoning in cooking, are fine to eat. The small amounts of salicylates contained in food and spices do not block guaifenesin.

As you now know, many cosmetics and toiletries, from toothpaste to sunscreens, contain enough salicylates to stop guaifenesin's therapeutic effects. Learning all of the plant and chemical names that indicate a salicylate may be present in a list of ingredients is not easy. Fortunately, there is a website where one can go to find lists of name brand products that are salicylate-free. The products listed include soaps, hair products, moisturizers, deodorants, toothpaste, razors (they must not contain an aloe strip or moisturizing strip), baby wipes, toners, cleansers, mosquito repellants, sunscreens, dental adhesives, makeup, acne skin care and just about aything else that is put on the body. The website address is: www.psha-inc.com/guai-support and click on the Sal-Free™ Centre.

Sal-Free™ is a trademarked name.

If you do not have a computer, most libraries have computers available and will show you how to go online. Use the above website to check the products that you already have at home and as a guide in choosing new products that are salicylate-free. This website also has a sal-free ingredient page where individual ingredients are listed if they do not contain salicylates. I do not recommend that you print the pages on this website as it is very long (more than 70 pages) and it is updated frequently due to new products and ingredient changes that companies make to existing products.

From time to time, companies may change some of the ingredients in their existing products without changing the name of the product. Sometimes the new ingredients contain salicylates. Once people begin using products that are salicylate-free, most will continue to use the same products thinking that they will remain salicylate-free, but this is not always true. Be sure to compare the ingredients of your newly purchased product with the ingredients from the old container you have at home to insure that none of the ingredients have changed and now contain salicylates. Return to the website from time to time to insure that products you have chosen are remaining salicylate-free. If you have a product that is not on the list of salicylate-free products, but it does not appear to contain any ingredients that contain salicylates, then go to the sal-free ingredient page and check each ingredient to make sure it is on this list.

Most prescription medications do not contain salicylates. Be sure and check with your pharmacy if you are not sure. However, any medication that is peppermint coated may block even if it does not contain aspirin. Nonprescription products are a different story and do frequently contain salicylates. Examples are Aspergum, Pepto Bismol and Ben Gay. There is a link from the sal-free product page to help guide you through salicylates in medications and supplements.

A conflict occurs when taking an aspirin a day for heart conditions. In most people, this amount of aspirin, even if it is a baby aspirin, will be a potent blocker. There are several solutions for this. You can ask your physician if it is possible for you to use a different medication that would have a similar effect. In some cases Coumadin, Ticlid, or Plavix may be appropriate. Another alternative is bromelain, a salicylate-free digestive enzyme that is a natural blood thinner.[3,4,5,6] If bromelain is being used in this way, it must be taken on an empty stomach. Depending on the person and the quality of the bromelain being used, it will usually take four to six bromelain to have the same blood thinning effect as one baby aspirin. A protime test can be done by your doctor that will monitor the blood thinning effect of whichever medication is chosen. The correct dose can then be determined from the protime results.

When changing products in your quest to become salicylate-free, take your time and be as thorough as possible. Some people who use very few products might be able to finish this process in several days while others who use a variety of cosmetics or supplements may need a full month or more. Once you are ready to start looking for possible sources of salicylates you may want to narrow your search down to just one area every several days. For example, take a day or two to investigate your entire collection of dental care products. This includes mouthwash, dental floss (no flavors allowed), toothpaste, breath mints, fluoride gel, denture cream, and so forth. Are your products on the salicylate-free web page? If not, pick out several products from that page and then go shopping to locate them. Salicylate-free toothpaste can be especially difficult to find, as can sunscreen. In many cases these products can be purchased from websites that specialize in salicylate-free products. After dental care products are scrutinized, you can then go to another category like makeup or vitamin supplements.

The initial salicylate elimination process is the hardest. In the future, you will just be replacing one or two products at a time and can check the product and the ingredients as you replace things.

8

Finding Your Dose

Finding your ideal dose of guaifenesin for treating the nonplus conditions can be a little tricky and requires patience, attention to symptoms, and persistence. Taking the optimum dose is important because too little guaifenesin results in no apparent improvement, and in most cases too much makes one feel consistently worse. *An extremely gradual dosing pattern improves chances of quickly finding the optimum dose and minimizing unnecessary exacerbations.*

Determining how many milligrams of guaifenesin to take each day should be done after you have eliminated all sources of salicylates that could block or partially block guaifenesin from working. Being completely salicylate free for about five days before using guaifenesin is a good idea and will help to determine if you are especially sensitive to salicylates. In people with greater salicylate sensitivity, this step of eliminating salicylates alone may result in some symptom improvement. Knowing if you are super salicylate sensitive can be helpful in making sure that you are especially vigilant about avoiding salicylates. If you are super salicylate sensitive, you will likely find that you must avoid even low salicylate items such as coffee and green tea to prevent aggravating some symptoms.

With any medication, taking the correct amount is critical for good results. There are a variety of ways to determine the proper dose of a medication based on several factors such as your size, symptom improvement, and achieving or improving a measurable goal such as bone density or red blood cell count. When using guaifenesin, I find that monitoring symptom changes and adjusting the dose until the optimum symptom changes occur most accurately finds the ideal dose. Size and weight do not seem to be significant factors in determining the ideal dose.

The basic procedure is to start at a low dose and each week increase the amount of guaifenesin you are taking by 200 to 300 mg (depending on the milligram content of the tablet you are taking), until you feel a significant change in your symptoms. This change may be a decrease in one or more symptoms, a temporary worsening of one or more symptoms, or most often, an improvement of some symptoms and at the same time a worsening of other symptoms.

Improvement of symptoms ranges from gradual to rapid, and in a small percentage of cases only mild improvements occur for the first several years. Some symptoms are likely to temporarily increase in intensity and frequency, but not beyond what you have already experienced. Because of this, you should continue to use any medication, supplements, and lifestyle aids that you are currently using that help you to manage pain and other problems, provided they are salicylate-free. Over time, most of my patients are able to decrease and even eliminate many or all of the drugs they once used to control symptoms. Remember, some drugs require a doctor's supervision to be safely lowered.

Guaifenesin has a low incidence of side effects, especially at the low doses usually taken by people treating nonplus conditions. Stomach discomfort is rare and usually mild. If this occurs it can usually be eliminated by taking guaifenesin with meals or placing the guaifenesin in a gelatin capsule. Allergic reaction is extremely rare, and I have never personally seen this occur. Because of the general lack of side effects, any increase in symptoms is almost always a result of guaifenesin reversing the processes that created the symptoms in the first place, and is not due to an adverse reaction. When a person who does not have a nonplus condition takes guaifenesin, there are no symptom changes other than those associated with guaifenesin's expectorant properties.

Many people are apprehensive about a possible increase in symptoms, so it is important to know that lowering the dose or even discontinuing guaifenesin temporarily can stop an increase in symptoms. In reality, changes are a good thing, even if some symptoms temporarily get worse, because it tells you that guaifenesin is working. In most cases, the symptoms that increase are a repeat of symptoms that are already present.

You may also intermittently experience symptoms that were present in the past but have been long forgotten. The sudden return of symptoms from the past is usually a positive sign that you are near the correct dose. Once the ideal dose is found, most people will experience at least intermittent symptomatic improvement within several weeks to one month, and many will have at least partial relief from problems that have been present for decades.

To know if a significant change in your symptoms is taking place, you must first be fully aware of all your different symptoms and their approximate frequency. Fill out the symptom summary sheet on page ix, at the beginning of the book, prior to starting guaifenesin. It lists many of the common symptoms associated with the nonplus conditions. Feel free to include additional symptoms you have experienced that you feel are a result of one or more of the nonplus conditions, but which are not included on the list of symptoms. You will use this chart to track symptom changes that occur once guaifenesin is started. The symptom summary sheet is necessary because when three or four or more symptoms are present at different frequencies of occurrence, it is easy to forget about the symptoms that have improved and thus not recognize that the correct dose has been reached.

Once you have eliminated salicylates and charted your symptoms, you should now be ready to start. Take 200 mg of quick-acting, (also known as immediate release) or 300 mg of long-acting, (also known as sustained release) guaifenesin in the morning and evening. Quick-acting guaifenesin often comes in 200, 300, and 400 mg tablets or capsules, so take whatever part is necessary to get the 200 mg dose that you will be starting with, morning and evening. Long-acting guaifenesin only comes in 600 mg pills. They are scored in the middle and are easy to break in half to get the 300 mg dose that you will take twice a day.

Once a long-acting guaifenesin pill is broken in half it will lose some of its long-acting characteristics, but this should not pose a problem when treating the nonplus conditions.

The starting total daily dose will be either 400 or 600 mg, depending on whether you are taking 200 mg or 300 mg twice a day. Continue this for one week. Be aware of any symptom changes that can occur in any of several ways. All or some symptoms could become temporarily worse in intensity or frequency. All or some symptoms could lesson with a decrease in frequency or intensity. The most common way for symptoms to change would be for some symptoms to decrease while at the same time other symptoms increase. There are also people who feel the changes in terms of good days (meaning much fewer symptoms than usual), and bad days (meaning that symptoms are the same or worse than usual). Another common indication that the guaifenesin is kicking in is the feeling of coming down with a cold or flu for several days. If this happens, continue taking the guaifenesin and the symptoms will usually stop in several hours or days. If by some coincidence you are actually getting a cold, guaifenesin will not be harmful. If the symptoms increase excessively, then decrease the dose as suggested in number 3 below.

After one week there should be three possible outcomes:

1. Little or no change would indicate that you are below the therapeutic dose, provided that you are not blocking with salicylates. We are looking for major changes in at least one or possibly several symptoms. Changes must be over and above your usual symptom variations in terms of frequency, intensity, and duration. Symptoms that increase could become as much of a problem as they have ever been in the past, and symptoms that decrease will become much less of a problem than what you have been commonly experiencing. If you are unsure whether or not significant changes have taken place there is no harm in continuing at the same dose for an additional week or more. If you decide that no significant changes have taken place, increase your daily dose by 200 or 300 mg, every week, until significant but tolerable changes take place.

2. Significant changes in the frequency or intensity of one or more symptoms. This may include improvement of some symptoms or worsening of some symptoms, and often a little of both. A significant change could also include the temporary return of a symptom that you have not experienced in many years. These are all signs that you are at or near your therapeutic dose. The dose that creates these types of changes should be the dose you continue to take.

3. A third possibility is an increase of symptoms that becomes too intense. The symptoms that increase are usually problems that are already being experienced or have been present in the past, but their frequency, duration, or intensity become intolerable. If this persists for a week it may indicate that too much guaifenesin is being taken. However, this is less likely to happen at the initial starting dose of 400 or 600 mg daily, since for most people this is the lowest therapeutic dose. If intolerable symptom changes do occur at the starting dose or at higher doses, there are several ways to handle this: A) Stop the guaifenesin completely for several days to a week. This will allow symptoms to return to their pre-guaifenesin status. Then resume at a dose 200 to 300 mg per day lower than what caused the intolerable symptoms. B) Continue taking guaifenesin but at a dose 200 to 300 mg lower, with half of the dose taken in the morning and half in the evening.

The dose that provides the greatest decrease in symptoms is the ideal dose. Even after finding your ideal dose, you may be able to fine-tune it with further small changes. If you feel better with an increase or decrease of 100 mg, then it may be good to remain at this dose. (A 100-mg dose is most easily achieved by breaking a 200-mg tablet in half.) For those people whose initial symptom changes do not include a decrease of symptoms, you should stay at the dose that gives a significant but tolerable increase of one or more symptoms. Usually within six weeks significant improvement of at least one symptom will begin.

Theoretically, according to the phosphate retention theory, a higher dose should increase the speed of recovery, but I have not found this to be true. There is no need to take a higher dose if it makes you feel consistently worse than your ideal dose. This ideal dose allows one to be relatively comfortable while working towards long-term recovery. As time goes on, gradual improvement continues, but can be interrupted sporadically by an increase of symptoms. It is not known why some symptoms improve rapidly while other symptoms may not improve for months or even years.

There is considerable latitude in the amount of guaifenesin that different people find effective. I have had patients find their ideal dose as low as 100 mg per day and as high as 3600 mg. When using quick-acting guaifenesin approximately 50 percent of my patients find their ideal dose at 400 milligrams per day while only about five percent need to take less than 400 mg. At 1200 mg per day, more than 90 percent have found their ideal dose.

Prior to November 2003, there were many brands of long-acting guaifenesin available. According to the FDA, a high percentage of the long-acting brands were not releasing properly and have been removed from the market. Because of this inconsistent quality, I had many patients who were unable to find an effective dose with some brands of the old long-acting guaifenesin, also known as extended-release. The FDA took action to eliminate this problem and now there are only several brands of single ingredient, extended release guaifenesin. One brand of guaifenesin has a combination of extended and immediate-release guaifenesin in one bi-layered tablet, but is usually referred to as extended release. Even with properly manufactured guaifenesin that is wholly or partly extended-release, it has been my experience that the average patient will find that their ideal dose is higher when compared to immediate-release guaifenesin. For example, I find about one half of the people using these types of guaifenesin will find 600 mg to be their ideal dose, and by 1800 mg around 90 percent will have reached their ideal dose.

The difference in dose between the time-released types of guaifenesin and non-timed-release guaifenesin should not be a problem as long as you are aware that your dose may be different if you change from one type to another. You may find you need to increase or decrease the dose that you have been taking to maintain the same level of symptom changes.

Sometimes the variable symptoms of the nonplus conditions together with the changes brought on by guaifenesin can be extremely confusing. This is why it is so important to chart your original symptoms and their typical frequency before starting on guaifenesin. Your goal is to find the dose where there is a significant but tolerable change in symptoms. When changing your dose, either up or down, give yourself at least a week to evaluate the effect of the new dose. Changing your dose every couple of days only leads to greater confusion.

If you are not feeling at least one area of improvement in the first month after finding what you thought was your ideal dose, only increased symptoms, then try to fine-tune your dose. A small increase or decrease of one-half or even one-fourth of a tablet might help. If you still are not feeling improvement, then stick with the dose that creates a tolerable increase in symptoms. Remain on this dose and be patient. In most cases, improvements will occur within several months, but in rare cases even longer.

After being on guaifenesin for several weeks, months, or even years, some people may feel that their initial improvements have gradually diminished or they have begun to feel consistently worse than before starting guaifenesin. This could be for a number of different reasons.

First, just in case, re-check all products you use for sources of salicylates that could be blocking. Eliminate any offending products.

Second, go to your symptom summary chart and make sure that you have not overlooked any key area of improvement. It is easy to focus on symptoms that increase or stay the same and forget about the symptoms that have become less troublesome or have been completely eliminated. If you realize that improvement has taken place, then continue at the same dose. It is much easier to put up with the symptoms that have worsened or that are remaining static when you are aware of other problems that have diminished. Regularly reviewing the symptom summary sheet reminds you what has improved and provides inspiration to continue.

If review of the symptom summary sheet confirms that initial improvements have diminished, and you have already determined that you are not blocking with salicylates, then a change in the guaifenesin dose may be necessary. If it appears that your symptoms are generally worse, a slight decrease in dose is recommended. If the symptoms are approximately the same as before guaifenesin was used, then increase the dose slightly. In these cases, the help of an experienced doctor may prove beneficial.

Lastly, there are many symptoms that can arise in our lives. Some are due to nonplus conditions, some arise from reversing these conditions with guaifenesin and some come from totally unrelated conditions. Symptoms such as chest pain, difficulty breathing, depression, vertigo, and others could be due to other causes and represent serious medical conditions, especially if you have not experienced these problems in relation to the nonplus conditions in the past. Once you start taking guaifenesin, do not assume that every symptom you experience is due to nonplus conditions or reversing the nonplus conditions with guaifenesin. It is important to seek medical attention if potentially serious symptoms occur. You need to be aware of what is happening with your body and seek medical attention when appropriate.

9

Reactive Hypoglycemia

Reactive hypoglycemia, sometimes known as carbohydrate intolerance or carbohydrate sensitivity, is a term that refers to a health condition in which blood sugar is lowered excessively several hours after eating a meal high in sugary or starchy carbohydrates. This is also sometimes called hypoglycemia, but this term is no longer considered appropriate under these circumstances. According to the National Institute of Diabetes and Digestive and Kidney Diseases, the symptoms associated with reactive hypoglycemia occur within four hours after eating.[1]

Understanding if you have reactive hypoglycemia and what to do about it is important because it is common for people to have both a nonplus condition and reactive hypoglycemia. These conditions can cause the same or very similar symptoms, which greatly complicates treatment unless reactive hypoglycemia is understood and properly addressed. Prior to using guaifenesin, I found that more people with a nonplus condition benefited from addressing this problem than any other single lifestyle change. Many physicians have concluded that reactive hypoglycemia can be considered a frequent co-condition of the nonplus conditions, particularly irritable bowel and chronic fatigue.

Reactive hypoglycemia is associated with meals or snacks high in starchy and/or sugary carbohydrates. A person who is sensitive to these types of carbohydrates will frequently experience symptoms, such as fatigue, extreme sleepiness, anxiety, and digestive complaints, when the body overreacts to these foods by secreting too much insulin. This oversecretion of insulin results in an excessively lowered blood sugar. This may seem strange, since sugars and starches are precisely the types of carbohydrates that can also rapidly raise blood sugar. It is true that carbohydrate will raise blood sugar, but in susceptible individuals sweet and starchy carbohydrates can also have the opposite result of lowering blood sugar several hours later in a type of rebound effect. There are varying degrees of sensitivity to carbohydrates, but in general, the more carbohydrates eaten at one time, the greater the insulin response and the greater the chance of lowered blood sugar and the symptoms associated with lowered blood sugar.

When explaining the cause of reactive hypoglycemia, the online Merck Manual states, "This is ascribed to a delayed and exaggerated rise in plasma insulin."[2] In other words, the body does not begin to release insulin quickly enough as the blood sugar begins to rise as a result of eating. This delay of the insulin response allows blood sugar to continue to rise, especially if the meal is high in carbohydrates. When the body finally does respond, the blood sugar has gone too high and results in an excessive release of insulin. Too much insulin has the result of lowering blood sugar too far. This low blood sugar is the cause of many symptoms including: sleepiness that can be extreme, dizziness, slow thinking, irritability, depression, headaches, excessive appetite, and strong cravings for junk food.

The body now needs to bring the low blood sugar back up to a normal level, and will usually do so in one of two ways. First, the body may respond with cravings for food that will rapidly raise blood sugar back up again. The foods that do this are sugary and starchy carbohydrates. Of course these foods will raise the blood sugar back up again, but if eaten to excess, they will also cause the same problem to return again. Thus, people who respond to low blood sugar by craving sweet and starchy carbohydrates recreate the problem over and over.

The second way for the body to bring the low blood sugar back up to normal is to release adrenaline. An adrenaline release will effectively raise blood sugar back up to normal levels but will also create unpleasant symptoms such as anxiety, a feeling of panic, nausea, sweating, digestive difficulty, gas, diarrhea, tight muscles, heart palpitations, and trouble sleeping.

High insulin levels may have one more harmful effect. Insulin lowers blood sugar by converting blood glucose into fat (lipid synthesis) while it works to prevent the burning of fat as a fuel (inhibits lipolysis). The combination of these two factors tends to cause weight gain with excessive carbohydrate intake.

All of these problems can often be avoided by reducing consumption of sugary and starchy carbohydrates that raise blood sugar rapidly. Some people have all the symptoms of reactive hypoglycemia and yet their doctors have told them that they do not have hypoglycemia because their blood sugar levels are not below 70mg/dl when tested. A study by medical researchers Genter and Ipp clearly showed that the symptoms of reactive hypoglycemia could occur when the blood sugar is considerably above 70mg/dl.[3] If you have the symptoms of reactive hypoglycemia after eating carbohydrates, and if eliminating the offending carbohydrates decreases or eliminates these symptoms, then you most likely do have reactive hypoglycemia, even if you technically do not have classic hypoglycemia.

Most people are simply unaware that carbohydrates can be the cause of so many health problems. Likewise, many doctors know very little about reactive hypoglycemia. Because of this lack of awareness, people can perpetuate these symptoms on a daily basis simply because of what they eat. As a consequence, the symptoms caused by reactive hypoglycemia can make it appear that guaifenesin is not working. Even if guaifenesin is doing its job, reactive hypoglycemia can continually cause fatigue, headaches, tight muscles, digestive upset, and other symptoms.

So, what is a carbohydrate? Carbohydrates as they relate to reactive hypoglycemia can be put into two categories, "good" and "bad." The "good" carbohydrates raise blood sugar very little and do not stimulate the body to release insulin. The "bad" carbohydrates quickly raise blood sugar, which may cause an exaggerated rise in insulin, followed by an excessive lowering of blood sugar.

Foods as diverse as doughnuts and celery are considered

carbohydrates. So, we must know the difference between the carbohydrates that cause the problems associated with reactive hypoglycemia and those that do not. The "bad" carbohydrates are sweet or starchy. The starchy carbohydrates include grains such as wheat products (crackers, breakfast cereals, bread, bagels, doughnuts, pasta), corn, rice, and potatoes. Incidentally, alcohol (which is made from grain or some other type of starchy carbohydrate) can also raise blood sugar. The sweet carbohydrates include naturally sweet foods like fruit, fruit juice and honey, as well as processed sweeteners, table sugar, corn syrup, fructose, molasses, and of course desserts, such as ice cream and cake. Most fresh fruit eaten in moderation does not raise blood sugar as much as one would think, but fruit juice, dried fruit, and very sweet fruit like grapes, bananas, and pineapple will raise blood sugar rapidly, unless eaten in small amounts.

Both sweet and starchy foods after being eaten and digested are rapidly converted to glucose. Glucose is released into the bloodstream in direct relationship to the amount of carbohydrate consumed. Once glucose is in the blood it is called blood sugar. It is the sudden rise of blood sugar that creates an over-secretion of insulin, resulting in reactive hypoglycemia. To effectively treat reactive hypoglycemia, one must restrict the sugary and starchy carbohydrates. In reality these carbohydrates are not truly bad unless they are eaten in excess. The problem is that what one person easily tolerates may be excessive for another.

Non-starchy vegetables like spinach, cabbage, and green beans are also a type of carbohydrate. Yet these non-starchy vegetables do not raise blood sugar or insulin in any significant amount. A more complete list of these very beneficial foods include tomatoes, onions, celery, all types of lettuce, bell peppers, greens, cucumbers, radishes, broccoli, mushrooms and raw carrots (cooked carrots do raise blood sugar and act more like a starch than a vegetable). These vegetables contain low amounts of sugar and starch but plenty of vitamins, minerals, and fiber. Fiber is a type of indigestible carbohydrate, also known as cellulose. Cellulose is not your typical carbohydrate, because it cannot be digested and it is not a source of calories. An indigestible carbohydrate is not converted to glucose but passes through the colon and is eliminated.

Reactive Hypoglycemia

Even though fiber is indigestible, most of us are aware of how important it is for optimal health and that most people need more fiber in their diet.

Some foods are combination foods. This means that they contain a combination of two or more of the following: carbohydrate, fat, protein, and fiber. Beans are a good example of this type of food. Beans contain a fair amount of protein, carbohydrate, and fiber. But not all beans are alike. Most canned beans contain added sugar and should be eaten in smaller portions. This is especially true of baked beans. Even without added sugar, some beans contain more carbohydrate than others. Pinto beans and garbanzo beans contain more carbohydrates than kidney, navy and fava beans. Nuts are another common combination food that contains fat, protein, and some carbohydrate. Like beans, some nuts contain much more carbohydrate than others. Compare labels when shopping and you will quickly see the differences. Generally, nuts without added sugar and eaten in moderation are acceptable and raise blood sugar only mildly.

Some foods that we think of as healthy may not be so healthy after all, especially if you have reactive hypoglycemia. Yogurt with fruit actually contains a large amount of sugar and is a poor choice. Unsweetened yogurt that has no added sugar is a better choice, and you can add some of your own fruit.

If you have the symptoms associated with reactive hypoglycemia, then you should try changing your diet by sharply decreasing sugary and starchy carbohydrates. If you do not feel that you have carbohydrate sensitivity, but you do suffer from irritable bowel, I recommend that you try decreasing your carbohydrates anyway. I find that most people with irritable bowel, or even a few digestive symptoms, often find remarkable improvement with a significant decrease in sugary and starchy foods. A good test is to completely eliminate these types of carbohydrates for two weeks. This means no sugar, grain, potatoes, corn, and alcohol. One-half to one piece of fruit three times per day with meals, or as a snack between meals, can be eaten—with the exception of bananas and dried fruit. Eat only small portions of the combination foods. With your carbohydrates greatly reduced, are you feeling better, having more energy, or having fewer digestive

71

complaints? You will discover that following this type of diet is not easy because strong cravings are common. If you cannot change your diet this drastically, then reduce your sweet and starchy carbohydrate intake as much as you can. It is likely that you will feel some improvement. The term carbohydrate addict comes from strong carbohydrate craving and is almost universal with reactive hypoglycemia. It is not easy to break the addiction, but those who do are amazed at how much better they feel. Fatigue, headaches, and possibly other symptoms are likely as your body throws a temper tantrum while you wean yourself off of carbohydrates.

After you have reduced your carbohydrate intake for two weeks, you may start adding small amounts of grains and fruit, one at a time, to determine how much carbohydrate you can tolerate before the symptoms of reactive hypoglycemia return. Eating smaller meals and adding a healthy snack between meals will help to stabilize blood sugar and decrease the amount of insulin released at meals. The order in which your food is eaten can also help you to be more successful at decreasing carbohydrate consumption. People tend to eat the carbohydrate portion of the meal first and then have little room for protein and vegetables. This is almost like eating dessert first. By reversing this order and eating the carbohydrates last you are likely to eat less carbohydrate. Frequent meals also help to control hunger and prevent a feeling of deprivation from setting in which may lead to binge eating.

Many popular diets recommend restricting sugary and starchy carbohydrates. Some of these are the Atkins Diet, the Zone, the G-Index Diet, the Schwarzbein Principle and the South Beach Diet. All of these diets recommend decreasing or eliminating sugary and starchy foods like sodas, candy, desserts, ice cream, bread, pasta, breakfast cereals, crackers, chips, rice, corn, potatoes, and almost any junk food. Following any of these diets will usually result in a decrease of symptoms caused by carbohydrate sensitivity, but some may not be strict enough for you to eliminate all of the symptoms. Carbohydrate sensitivity varies greatly from person to person. A carbohydrate that does not bother one person may put another person into a tailspin. This is why it is best to just eliminate all sweet and starchy carbohydrates for two weeks, and then gradually add carbohydrates to see what you can and cannot tolerate.

Sugary and starchy foods form the basis of most peoples' diets. Think of the average breakfast: cereal, toast, and juice. This is basically carbohydrate, carbohydrate, carbohydrate, with only a little protein coming from the milk in the cereal. This overdependence on carbohydrates is common at most meals, partly because carbohydrates are convenient and inexpensive, and partly because we love the way they taste. When carbohydrates are decreased, it only makes sense that you will be eating more vegetables, proteins, and fats. Be willing to try something new. Vegetables of the non-starchy variety mentioned above are good choices and there are many more that I did not mention, from kohlrabi to scallop squash.

Protein sources include meat (eat smaller portions of sugar-cured meats), poultry, fish, eggs, and cottage cheese. If you do not like the idea of eating a lot of meat, find a quality source of protein powder that does not contain added sugar. Protein powder can come from soy, egg, whey, rice, and other sources, so you have a lot to choose from. Fat sources are olives and olive oil, avocado, flax meal, nuts, and moderate amounts of dairy, such as cheese and sour cream. For many people the cravings for carbohydrates will be strong, but focus on what you can eat and how much better you are feeling.

10

Frequently asked questions

Q: Can you prove that guaifenesin effectively treats the nonplus conditions?

A: I can say that not only have I proved it for myself, but thousands of people who are taking guaifenesin are also convinced. Proving it through a controlled trial, however, is expensive and this type of proof is not likely to occur anytime soon. Guaifenesin is a generic compound, making it unlikely that a pharmaceutical company would be willing to spend the millions of dollars that it would take to do a trial. Furthermore, a controlled clinical trial is not always more accurate than a doctor's clinical experience. Many people and doctors have witnessed phenomenal changes using guaifenesin, and I am confident that studies will eventually reflect this reality. Unfortunately, there are many difficulties associated with performing a formal study of the nonplus conditions. These include the lack of objective findings by which to judge guaifenesin's effectiveness, and the necessity of tracking dozens of possible symptoms. In addition to these problems, guaifenesin as a treatment will be especially difficult to study, because of the great variability in what constitutes an ideal dose and salicylate sensitivity differences between people. There are also differences in the initial response to guaifenesin, with some people feeling better, some worse, and most people feeling worse in some areas and better in others.

The overdependence on randomized clinical trials is one of the primary points of Dr. James Le Fanu's award-winning and critically acclaimed book, *The Rise and Fall of Modern Medicine*. In discussing the weaknesses of the randomized controlled trial, his book states, "...sometimes—perhaps even often—the 'clinical wisdom' of doctors assessing the efficacy of treatment based on their own personal experience may, after all, be a better guide to medical practice than 'the objectivity' of the clinical trial." He continues, "They are, it is argued, insufficiently sensitive to variations in the range of symptoms of disease and thus the responsiveness to treatment."[1]

I cannot think of any conditions that have greater numbers of symptoms, or greater ranges in the variation of symptoms, than the nonplus conditions. This would indicate that a clinical trial for the nonplus conditions might be especially difficult in terms of producing trustworthy conclusions.

Q: How is it possible for guaifenesin to treat the dozens and possibly hundreds of symptoms associated with conditions discussed in this book?

A: It is not uncommon for one health condition to cause many different symptoms. When the cause of the condition is addressed, all of the related symptoms will usually resolve. This is true for the nonplus conditions, just as it is for other conditions. The disease scurvy, although now rare, is an example of a condition that is responsible for a wide variety of symptoms. Scurvy can cause weakness, anemia, spongy and bleeding gums, hardening of the muscles in the legs, increased susceptibility to infections and many other symptoms. We now know that scurvy and all of the wide-ranging symptoms it causes are the result of a vitamin C deficiency. When the diet contains vitamin C in great enough amounts, all of the symptoms of scurvy are eliminated. It was noted by several individuals that certain foods, especially oranges, lemons, and limes, were of value in treating scurvy by the early 1600s.[2] For reasons that are not completely clear, this curative treatment was not generally recognized as being useful until the mid-1800s. For some inexplicable reason, groups of doctors even organized against using fruit as a treatment for scurvy. It was not until 1918 that vitamin C, the ingredient in citrus that eliminates scurvy, was discovered.

Scurvy is comparable to the nonplus conditions in several ways.

1. Both scurvy and the nonplus conditions can cause a wide variety of confusing symptoms.
2. Effective treatments for scurvy and the nonplus conditions are available that treat all of the symptoms. (I am not saying that guaifenesin is 100 percent effective for every individual with nonplus conditions, as vitamin C is for scurvy.)
3. Effective treatment for scurvy existed before there was an understanding of what vitamin C was or how it helped, just as guaifenesin is an effective treatment for the nonplus conditions, in spite of the fact that how it works is not fully understood.

Q: I desperately want to try guaifenesin due to severe fibromyalgia, irritable bowel, and interstitial cystitis, but I am afraid because I might feel worse before I feel better. There is no way I can tolerate feeling any worse. What should I do?

A: Starting guaifenesin makes most people feel a little anxious because no one wants to feel worse. In most cases, when you do experience symptoms that increase, they may intermittently become worse than what you experience on average, but not worse than what they have ever been. Having pain exceed what it has been in the past could be a sign that you have gone beyond your therapeutic dose of guaifenesin. The first month of taking guaifenesin at a therapeutic dose is frequently the time of most intense symptom increase. There is also a possibility that the symptom changes will entail a substantial reduction of intensity or frequency.

For most people who are anxious about guaifenesin, starting at a low dose and very gradually increasing the dose as necessary, relieves their anxiety. It is also a comfort to know that at any time you can simply stop the guaifenesin, and it will be out of your system within about 24 hours. The plasma half-life for guaifenesin is one hour, although no one knows how long guaifenesin remains on receptor sites.[3]

Q: Is all guaifenesin the same? Does all guaifenesin work equally well when treating chronic fatigue or fibromyalgia?

A: Single-ingredient guaifenesin refers to a product where guaifenesin is the only active ingredient. This is the only guaifenesin I recommend for the nonplus conditions. Guaifenesin that is combined with other ingredients, whether in cough syrups or in pill form, is not generally considered appropriate for our purposes.

Single-ingredient guaifenesin comes in two types, both of which are non-prescription: immediate-release guaifenesin, IR, and extended-release, ER, guaifenesin. Immediate-release guaifenesin is also called QA, meaning quick-acting, and FA, fast-acting. Immediate-release guaifenesin is also available as a liquid and is found in most grocery and drug stores. The liquid form frequently contains food coloring and sweeteners and is not recommended for long-term use due to these additives. Guaifenesin contained in liquid cough and cold medications is also not considered appropriate for treating the nonplus conditions, due to the other ingredients. Extended-release guaifenesin is known by several other names: long acting, LA, and sustained-release, SR, and bi-layered.

The two different types of single ingredient guaifenesin currently sold work well when used for treating the nonplus conditions. However, if a person changes the type of guaifenesin used (from immediate-release to extended-release or vice versa), an adjustment in dose may be necessary to achieve the same level of symptomatic change. It is not unusual to require a slightly lower daily dose if one is using immediate-release, when compared to extended-release. Conversely, an increased dose may be necessary if switching from immediate-release to extended-release. The difference in dose between the two often ranges from 20 percent to 70 percent. However, a change in dose is not always required. If you change from one type to another, pay attention to your symptom changes and be prepared to alter your dose to achieve the ideal amount of symptomatic change, as discussed in Chapter 8, *Finding Your Dose*.

Because of problems with the release rate of many brands of extended-release guaifenesin, the FDA has stopped all companies except one from selling it. After December of 2003, the only single-ingredient extended release guaifenesin available was a bi-layered guaifenesin that contains some immediate-release guaifenesin also. This product is labeled as an extended release guaifenesin and the above suggestions for extended-release still apply. Since 2005, additional companies have been allowed to sell extended release guaifenesin.

Even though all brands of guaifenesin currently available work consistently well, whether extended-release or immediate-release, you should be aware that many brands of extended-release guaifenesin sold prior to December 2003 may not be effective.[4] This unfortunate problem has no doubt resulted in many people and physicians failing to get results when using it as a treatment for the nonplus conditions. If you were one of the people who used ER, SR, or LA guaifenesin before December 2003 and did not get the results expected, I encourage you to give guaifenesin another try.

Q: I hear some people talking about FDA-approved guaifenesin. Are there some brands of guaifenesin that are not FDA-approved?

A: All legally manufactured single-ingredient guaifenesin, whether immediate-release or extended-release, is FDA-approved. According to the FDA no approval by them has a higher status than another, with regards to guaifenesin.[5]

Q: My doctor tells me that the only thing guaifenesin does is thin mucus, and that he does not understand how it could help all of the conditions that you claim it can. He also says that the doses you find effective are too low to do anything.

A: Fortunately, doctors and researchers are continually finding beneficial new uses for existing medications. There are many examples of compounds, long used for one purpose, being later discovered to be helpful for completely different conditions. For example, methotrexate was initially used to treat malignancy. Many years later it was discovered to treat several types of arthritic conditions. For malignancy it must be used intravenously and in high doses, but for the arthritic conditions it can be taken orally and is effective at a much lower dose. Because of methotrexate's effectiveness with different conditions and different doses, doctors believe that there could be several modes of action that this drug has in the body.[6] Even though no one can explain how methotrexate works for these completely dissimilar conditions, it is used simply because it is effective. It would seem that guaifenesin also has more than one mode of action in the body and works in a wide range of milligram amounts.

Q: Some people use the procedure known as mapping to determine dose, but you recommend using symptoms. Why? (Please see page 39 for the explanation on mapping.)

A: It has been suggested by Dr. St. Amand that mapping, in addition to providing confirmation of the diagnosis of the nonplus conditions, can be used to determine when the therapeutic dose of guaifenesin has been reached. An initial map is made reflecting the lumps and bumps that can be felt on the body. Guaifenesin is then taken and gradually increased until the lumps and bumps diminish in size and/or number, when compared to the original map. Mapping is performed every one to four weeks and the dose is gradually increased until the map improves. The dose at which the map improves is considered to be the therapeutic dose.[7]

I have been unable to resolve several contradictory factors associated with using mapping to determine dose. As a part of his phosphate retention theory, Dr. St. Amand believes that water enters cells as the body begins to remove stored phosphate due to taking guaifenesin. This water increases the size of the lumps and bumps for a time.[8] I tend to agree with this because I commonly find that as a result of taking guaifenesin, the lumps and bumps do increase in size, and this can persist for more than a year. However, this is contradictory to the concept of mapping, which is contingent upon guaifenesin reducing the lumps and bumps. I also find that the lumps and bumps may remain unchanged for many months, even when the patient is feeling greatly recovered. Only approximately one-third of my patients have an immediate decrease in the lumps and bumps that coincides with significant symptom changes.

Although there are some people who are using mapping in this way to determine dosage, I do not believe that it is the easiest, fastest, or most effective way. That is why I primarily use symptom changes to determine dosage and employ mapping more as a diagnostic aid.

Finally, if mapping was an accurate way to determine dose, the problems with extended release guaifenesin should have been discovered many years before I noticed this problem by using symptoms as a guide for dosing.

Q: I still have a long swelling in the front of my left thigh after five months of being on guaifenesin. I have heard that once I am at the correct dose this swelling should clear after the first month, but mine has not. What should I do?

A: If you have decided to use changes in the lumps and bumps to determine dose, I cannot tell you what to do, since I believe this to be a confusing and inaccurate method to find the ideal dose of guaifenesin. If you decide to use symptom changes to determine dosage, I recommend you ignore the left thigh. In my experience the left thigh has no more significance than any other part of the body when it comes to the lumps and bumps. I have many patients with one of the nonplus conditions who have never had lumps, bumps, or swellings in the left thigh at all, just as some people do not have lumps, bumps, or swellings in their arms, abdomen, or calf muscles. If the left thigh was an accurate way to determine at what dose guaifenesin is effective, then this method should have found that many brands of sustained-released were not working properly. Yet, no one using the left thigh as an indicator for dosing could tell when a brand of guaifenesin was or was not working.

Q: I would like to use one of the aquarium phosphate testing kits to determine if guaifenesin is helping me to eliminate phosphate. Will this be accurate?

A: No. This test equipment is made for aquariums, not people. If you want to test your urinary excretion of phosphate you must perform a

24-hour urine phosphate study through a reputable laboratory. To determine if your excretion of phosphate is higher with guaifenesin, you need to collect urine from every voiding during a 24-hour period. Then this would need to be compared to another 24-hour period where you collected all of your urine and were not using guaifenesin.

I have done 24-hour urine phosphate studies on myself while not taking guaifenesin, and others while taking guaifenesin. I have completed a total of six of these tests. Four of the tests were done while taking guaifenesin, but only one of these test showed an increased excretion of phosphate when compared to the tests that were done while not on guaifenesin. Several other research studies had come up with similar findings. This is why I state that the phosphate excretion theory may not stand the test of time. However, after being on guaifenesin since the year 2000, I am 90 percent recovered. The fact that guaifenesin does work is much more important than how it works.

Q: I have been taking guaifenesin for three weeks and have eliminated all salicylates. I am waiting for an increase in pain and fatigue, but instead I am experiencing noticeably less pain and more energy. If I am at the correct dose, shouldn't I be feeling worse?

A: Absolutely not! Not everyone has an increase in the severity or frequency of symptoms. Thinking that the therapeutic dose requires one to feel worse, in my opinion, is a major fallacy associated with guaifenesin treatment. I have seen many people who felt improvement at a particular dose, but continued to raise their dose until they were miserable, thinking that they were doing the right thing. Taking more than what is needed will make almost anyone with the nonplus conditions feel worse. Feeling terrible is neither necessary, nor is it our goal. The goal of using guaifenesin is to feel better, while at the same time treating the underlying cause of the condition. The ideal dose will do this. It is determined by a significant but tolerable change of symptoms. It has been my experience (rare exceptions are discussed below) that once a person has reached the therapeutic dose, symptoms change initially in one of four ways:

1. A significant decrease in some symptoms.
2. Some symptoms increase while other symptoms decrease.
3. A significant but tolerable increase in symptoms, including the feeling of coming down with a cold or flu for several days.
4. Alternating good days where most symptoms are decreased, and bad days where most symptoms are the same or increased.

I believe that the second scenario is the most common and best describes what initially occurs in the majority of people. As a person remains on a therapeutic dose, chances are that the patient will eventually experience several of the different ways that symptoms change.

Q: If guaifenesin is as effective as you and others claim, then why haven't other doctors reported similar beneficial effects?

A: Actually, more than 200 years ago, guaiac, which comes from the guaiacum tree, was used extensively to treat rheumatism.[9] The synthesized version of guaiac is now called guaifenesin. For centuries, rheumatism has been and remains a catchall term that primarily refers to gout, osteoarthritis, rheumatoid arthritis and fibromyalgia. Guaiac was one of the treatments found to have some merit in the treatment of rheumatism. We now know that guaiac is not helpful for arthritis or gout. It is reasonable to believe that it must have been helping those with fibromyalgia and the other nonplus conditions, just as guaifenesin does today.

Two things happened around the turn of the 19th century that would have a profound effect on guaiac and later guaifenesin as an effective treatment for fibromyalgia. It was during this time that salicylates in the form of ground willow bark had become the standard drug for the treatment of arthritis. Then, in 1897, acetylsalicylic acid (ASA) was synthesized and aspirin was born. It was also at this time that personal hygiene was improving, not just with clean water and indoor plumbing, but with increased availability of soaps, perfume and other toiletries, skin care products and the like, which commonly contain salicylates. These products were becoming more available to all classes of people.

With salicylate use from a variety of sources becoming so common, guaiac, and later guaifenesin, was no longer consistently effective when treating fibromyalgia, chronic fatigue, or irritable bowel. However, the increase in salicylate use had no detrimental effect on the ability of guaifenesin to thin mucus secretions. Consequently, loosening mucus secretions appeared to be the only benefit that guaiac or guaifenesin appeared to be giving.

Another factor, which greatly complicates the treatment of the nonplus conditions, is reactive hypoglycemia. One hundred years ago, white flour, sugar, junk food, and overeating were much less common. With these foods largely absent from the average person's diet, reactive hypoglycemia was much less common. Without the complications of reactive hypoglycemia the positive effects from guaiac would be more easily noticed.

With blocking due to salicylate use less likely, and reactive hypoglycemia almost unheard of, the primary stumbling blocks associated with guaifenesin in modern times were not prevalent in the early history of guaiac's use. Thus, in the 1800's and earlier, one may have been more likely to see the benefits of guaiac when used on people with fibromyalgia and the other nonplus conditions. I am sure there are a multitude of other reasons why the effects of guaiac (and later guaifenesin) have been overlooked, and I believe a book could be written on that topic alone.

In Chapter 1, I explained how I meet about two to four people per year who on their own have accidentally discovered that guaifenesin greatly decreases their symptoms that are associated with nonplus conditions. These people are surprised to find that other people are using it for similar problems. I meet these people after they hear about the guaifenesin support group that meets in my office. They attend a meeting out of curiosity and a desire to find out more about this treatment. No doubt these are people who happen to use products with very few salicylates or are not particularly sensitive to blocking with salicylates. Many of these people have also discovered on their own that several products, such as aloe and aspirin, prevent guaifenesin from being effective. Unfortunately, the numbers of people who have been lucky enough to discover guaifenesin on their own are so insignificant that few doctors have ever come across such people.

Q: I do not seem to notice any difference or changes in my symptoms, regardless of the amount of guaifenesin that I take. What should I do?

A: The first thing to think of is blocking, which can occur regardless of the dose of guaifenesin taken. In some cases blocking is not the problem. There is a small percentage of people whose symptoms do not change significantly for several months and even up to a year or more, even when taking what I consider to be high doses of guaifenesin, 2400 milligrams and greater. When this happens one can stay at a high dose, with approval of their doctor, until symptoms start to change. This requires a considerable amount of patience, but most people are eventually rewarded with gradual improvements. Once obvious symptom changes begin, monitor the changes to determine the best dose, as discussed in Chapter 8.

Alternatively, one can find someone who maps and attempt to determine the dose at which the lumps and bumps start to change. When using mapping for this purpose I believe that a sudden increase in the lumps may be a more common finding initially than a decrease, yet either change may indicate the correct dose has been reached.

Q: Do I really have to give up all of my personal care products that contain salicylates?

A: If you want the best possible chance of guaifenesin working for you, then the answer is yes. It is very hard to experience consistent improvement of symptoms when blocking with salicylates. However, it is usually acceptable to block for short periods of time. It is believed that in most cases salicylates remain in the system no longer than twenty-four hours following their use. Because of this, the occasional use of products that block should not pose a problem for most people. Examples include a day at the beauty salon, or use of an herbal product like echinacea for several days to head off a cold. If you do this from time to time, continue to use guaifenesin on these days. Since there is no way to know how much guaifenesin is actually blocked, you might as well take your usual amount of guaifenesin.

Being cautious with salicylates is always the best policy. Whether from intentional or unintentional salicylate use, my staff and I have seen many people slam their progress to a halt by using the wrong hairspray, sunscreen, or other product. Many patients have come to the office in tears from pain and frustration without a clue as to what has gone wrong until the offending blocker has been detected.

Q: If I am at the wrong dose, will all of that time have been wasted?

A: The premise of this question is based upon the phosphate retention theory. According to this theory, guaifenesin increases the excretion of phosphates that are being abnormally stored in the body. If this theory is true, even a little guaifenesin increases the excretion of phosphates, which is a good thing. However, until one is at the therapeutic dose, a significant decrease in phosphates may not occur. It is theorized that if one is taking a dose above the optimum therapeutic dose, then the phosphates are being eliminated at an accelerated rate. This is good if true, but it generally occurs at the cost of greatly increased symptoms.

If your dose of guaifenesin has been too low, it is likely that this dose has depleted some phosphate storage and this is positive. Also, at this time you were learning about salicylates and other details of using guaifenesin that will serve you well later.

Q: What does it feel like to block with salicylates?

A: Salicylates prevent guaifenesin from working, so if salicylates are blocking guaifenesin a variety of problems can arise. If blocking occurs while you are trying to find your proper dose of guaifenesin, you may find that ever-higher doses of guaifenesin have little or no effect. If you start blocking after you have already found your therapeutic dose, then how you feel with blocking depends upon how guaifenesin is changing your symptoms at that particular time. For example, if using guaifenesin has resulted in improved sleep, but has also aggravated your back pain, blocking could cause a return of sleep problems and less back pain.

Most of the time blocking makes a person feel like they were before guaifenesin was started. Blocking may not be immediately apparent; it may take several days or a week to feel the effects of blocking, depending on the individual or the amount of salicylate exposure. If the blocking is only partial, or salicylate exposure only occurs every several days, realizing that blocking is taking place can take even longer.

As you can see, blocking adds another layer of confusion to an already complicated process. There is a trick one can use to determine if blocking is occurring. Most people who take more guaifenesin than their therapeutic dose will feel a significant increase in symptoms over and above what was commonly experienced prior to using guaifenesin. If you can increase your dose by one pill for several days without feeling worse, then you might be blocking. If you are not blocking, then this increase will likely result in an increase in symptoms.

Q: I no longer feel like I am improving; could I be blocking?

A: When several symptoms are remaining troublesome month after month, people may feel they are no longer progressing. This could be due to the issues that we have already discussed: blocking with salicylates, a dose that is actually a little too high or too low for consistent symptom progress; a change in guaifenesin brands or types that require a dose change; and lastly, you may have started using one of the older brands of extended-release guaifenesin that does not release properly. Many times however, this static feeling is just a temporary lull in symptom changes that almost everyone experiences from time to time. This is sometimes referred to as stalling.

First, go to your symptom review sheet. Can you identify symptoms that remain substantially improved or completely eliminated? If yes, then you may not be blocking. Continue at your current dose, be patient, and continue to be aware of any potential sources of salicylates. For the majority of people, it can take many years to significantly improve every symptom. It is not uncommon for some symptoms to remain unchanged for years while others improve quickly and still others are present at a reduced level. Most people have had nonplus symptoms for many years. During this time, people are not feeling worse every single day. It is common to experience months or years where some symptoms remain roughly the same. When using guaifenesin, there will also be long stretches of time where the symptoms become stationary. As long as the improvements that have already occurred do not seem to be reversing, it is often best to remain at the same dose.

You may find that, yes, some symptoms had definitely changed for a period of many weeks or months, but they now seem to be returning to join the symptoms that never did change. This indicates that salicylates may be blocking, but could also be the result of a change in types or brands of guaifenesin. Changing types or brands may require that you slightly change your dose up or down to maintain the same level of symptom change.

If after reviewing your original symptom list you find that no significant symptom changes have actually taken place, then it is likely you were never at your therapeutic dose. Sometimes it is easy to believe that changes are taking place when they are actually just the usual fluctuation of symptoms experienced with the nonplus conditions. At this point, an increase in guaifenesin would be indicated. A variation on this is, "Yes, all of my symptoms have changed, but overall they have changed for the worse." If this is true for a period of several weeks or months, then this is a strong indicator that too much guaifenesin is being taken.

Q: Taking guaifenesin has made me feel worse; what should I do?

A: It is normal for some symptoms to increase once your therapeutic dose has been reached. Within a month, however, other symptoms should be decreasing or you should be experiencing occasional days of considerable relief where some symptoms are greatly reduced. If after several weeks, you have only experienced a worsening of symptoms, then it is likely that you are taking too much guaifenesin. Remember, some people improve on as little as 100 milligrams per day, although this is rare. In other instances increasing by 200 or 300 milligrams may be too much of an increase. For example, a person may not notice any changes at 400 milligrams of guaifenesin daily. When the dose is increased to 600 milligrams, everything feels worse and stays worse.

In this case a solution could be to increase by only 100 milligrams, for a daily dose of 500 milligrams. This is why I believe it is best to start with 200 milligram tablets.

If you suspect that your dose is too high, you can go about finding your ideal dose several ways. Start reducing your dose gradually until you find the ideal dose. The other way is to stop guaifenesin completely for several days to a week, and then start at a considerably lower dose than what was causing the increased symptoms. Gradually increase your guaifenesin dose until you notice the appropriate symptom changes.

Q: I have had chronic fatigue and irritable bowel since I was a child; shouldn't I be on a higher dose than most people?

A: Dose is neither determined by the length of time you have had any one of these conditions, nor by their severity. Neither is dose influenced by one's weight or sex. In most instances an effective dose is most easily and accurately found by symptom changes.

Q: I had just started taking guaifenesin when I suddenly started having the symptoms of a cold. Could this be due to guaifenesin?

A: Cold-like symptoms could indicate that you are coming down with something. It can be dangerous to assume that every symptom that comes along is due to the changes that guaifenesin can cause. Taking guaifenesin does not make one immune to other health conditions, such as pneumonia, heart problems, or ulcers. Use the same judgment that you would have used before taking guaifenesin, when it comes to seeing a doctor for symptoms. That being said, it is not unusual for the feelings of a cold or flu to come on for several days shortly after taking the dose of guaifenesin that is therapeutic for you.

If you are coming down with a cold or flu, guaifenesin can continue to be taken. In fact, many cough syrups contain guaifenesin to thin mucus secretions and make coughs more productive. If you do take a cough syrup that contains guaifenesin, remember to adjust your daily dose accordingly.

Q: Lately I have been experiencing numbness in my fingers and arms. Could this be from guaifenesin activating old symptoms?

A: Yes, it could be, but it could also be from a variety of other medical conditions. I will repeat the recommendation made in the answer above. Use the same judgment that you would have used before taking guaifenesin when it comes to seeing a doctor for symptoms.

Q: I've read that hormone imbalances are the cause of chronic fatigue, especially thyroid and estrogen.

A: Thyroid problems and female hormone imbalances cause many symptoms, but they do not cause any of the nonplus conditions. Hormone problems should receive appropriate treatment. It is possible and relatively common for a person to have one or more of the nonplus conditions as well as a hormone imbalance.

Q: I've heard that most people with fibromyalgia, irritable bowel and chronic fatigue are overachievers or Type A personalities.

A: I do not believe that people with the nonplus conditions are more likely to be Type A than the rest of the population. There are also people who believe that chronic fatigue sufferers are just lazy and want attention. This belief has no more validity than the Type A theory. As far as we can tell, people with chronic fatigue and the other nonplus conditions are as varied as the general population. Some have cancer, some are lazy or overachievers, while others suffer from PMS (pre-menstrual syndrome), or high blood pressure.

Q: What is the relationship between fibromyalgia and trigger points/ myofascial pain?

A: I believe that these are two different conditions that can produce similar symptoms; much like low thyroid and chronic fatigue can cause similar symptoms, but are unrelated. Unfortunately, trigger points and myofascial pain cannot be ruled out with medical tests, as thyroid problems often can be. This leaves differentiating trigger points/ myofascial pain and fibromyalgia to subtle differences in the pain, response to treatments, and other clues.

In general, the pain from fibromyalgia is more widespread throughout the body, migratory in nature, and frequently waxes and wanes more than the pain associated with trigger points. Some authorities have suggested that myofascial pain is a localized form of fibromyalgia, however, I disagree.[10] Myofacial and trigger-point therapy has progressed significantly since the early 1980's and has resulted in much more effective treatments for these problems, and often resolves them. This contrasts with the pain associated with fibromyalgia, which only temporarily responds to these treatments, if at all. In many instances fibromyalgia, trigger points and myofascial pain can occur in the same individual. In these cases a combination of structural and soft tissue treatment, along with guaifenesin, will have the maximum benefit.

11

Defining the Nonplus Conditions

- Chronic Fatigue and Immune Dysfunction Syndrome
- Ehlers-Danlos Syndrome
- Fibromyalgia
- Interstitial Cystitis
- Irritable Bowel Syndrome
- Multiple Chemical Sensitivity
- Neurally Mediated Hypotension
- Restless Legs Syndrome
- Vulvodynia

This chapter contains a description of each nonplus condition in alphabetical order. I have not attempted to give a detailed description of every single aspect of these conditions, but merely a general overview of generally accepted facts regarding these conditions.

To review, these conditions commonly occur together, share many symptoms and have the same basic characteristics. The cause or causes of all of these conditions are unknown, they are difficult to diagnose due to the lack of positive medical findings, are resistant to conventional treatment, but usually respond favorably to guaifenesin therapy. Some of these conditions cause just one type of symptom, such as restless legs syndrome, while fibromyalgia and chronic fatigue can potentially cause dozens of different symptoms that can extend far beyond the body pain or fatigue that their names imply. I have seen every one of these conditions resolve with the use of guaifenesin. This does not mean that in every single instance guaifenesin will be beneficial, for few treatments are 100 percent effective. It is possible that some of these conditions have more than one cause, and not all of these causes will respond to guaifenesin.

There are several additional conditions that I believe may be eventually added to this list. These conditions include Primary Raynaud's, pelvic pain syndromes, Gulf War Syndrome and periodic limb movement disorder which is similar to restless legs. I do not have enough experience treating patients with these conditions to include them at this time.

Chronic Fatigue Syndrome (CFS) and Chronic Fatigue with Immune Dysfunction Syndrome (CFIDS)

Chronic Fatigue and Chronic Fatigue with Immune Dysfunction Syndrome are complex, chronic illnesses that can negatively affect multiple body systems. Common problems include low energy, difficulty sleeping, poor memory, inability to think clearly, and mood disorders. Some people with chronic fatigue also experience frequent cold and flu-like symptoms, possibly due to some type of immune dysfunction, hence the two names.

Although its name trivializes the illness as seeming to be little more than tiredness, chronic fatigue with or without immune dysfunction syndrome can also cause the following symptoms, often with a wide range in frequency and severity.

- Extreme fatigue following even mild physical activity or exercise.
- Impairment of thought, speech, reasoning, and comprehension sometimes known as fog.
- Difficulties with eyes such as burning, blurring, and sensitivity to light.
- Mood changes including depression and irritability
- Dizziness and balance problems.

- Sensitivity to heat, cold, or sound
- Irregular heartbeat; pressure in the chest, throat, jaw and chest pain
- Unexplained fevers, feeling of a constant low grade fever, or low body temperature.
- Painful and swollen lymph nodes.
- Sore throat; constant throat clearing, and tingling or pulling in throat.
- Creepy crawly feelings and or burning sensations on the skin and rashes/ itching.

The majority of people with CFS and CFIDS concurrently experience one or more of the nonplus conditions, such as fibromyalgia, irritable bowel, neurally mediated hypotension, and multiple chemical sensitivities.[1]

Diagnosis of chronic fatigue can be a time-consuming and difficult process, which is generally arrived at by excluding other illnesses with similar symptoms, and comparing a patient's symptoms with the symptoms commonly attributed to chronic fatigue. Complicating the diagnostic process, people with CFS and CFIDS have symptoms that vary considerably from person to person, and frequently fluctuate in severity. Symptoms may come and go for no reason, while others may remain constant. Most symptoms cannot be seen, making it difficult for others to understand or believe the vast array of debilitating symptoms.[2] The cause or causes have not yet been identified and no specific diagnostic tests are available that can clearly identify the disorder.[3]

Because of the lack of positive tests and the fact that a person with chronic fatigue often looks fine, they may be accused of needing attention, being depressed, or malingering. Sufferers are often acutely aware that their symptoms "do not make sense," and may eventually believe they are just stressed, depressed, or "different." For unknown reasons, symptoms can be increased during times of stress (emotional, physical, or chemical) and during a woman's menstrual cycle, but are just as likely to wax and wane for no reason at all.

Likewise, symptoms of CFS and CFIDS may initially begin after a minor illness such as a cold or flu, after a period of high stress, or for no reason at all. For unknown reasons CFS is diagnosed two to four times more often in women that in men. Since no cause for CFS has been identified, (infectious agents in particular have been extensively investigated, but no association has been found), treatment programs are directed at relief of symptoms, with the goal of the patient regaining some level of pre-existing function and well being.

There are several unrelated health conditions that may cause similar symptoms: lupus, hypothyroidism, and Lyme's disease. These and other possible conditions should be ruled out, or if present, treated.

A study conducted by researchers at DePaul University showed that CFS is many times more common than previously believed and occurs across all ethnic groups and income levels.[4] Research published in 2001 indicates that CFS is more common among identical twins (who share the same genes) than fraternal twins (who share only some genes). Inheritance, then, may play a role in many cases.[5]

Ehlers-Danlos Syndrome (EDS)

EDS results from a defect in connective tissue, the tissue that provides support and connects parts of the body together. The root of the problem is faulty collagen, a protein that acts as glue, adding strength and elasticity to connective tissue. Tendons and ligaments are two types of connective tissue that are commonly affected by EDS. This condition may cause any of the following symptoms[6]:

- Fragile or stretchy rubber band-like skin
- Skin that bruises or scars easily and slow wound healing
- Loose, unstable joints prone to pain and misalignment
- Mitral valve prolapse
- Hiatal hernia
- Harmless bumps under the skin
- Some types of EDS can affect organs as well.

A major problem is that a person can look well, so is not taken seriously when complaining of joint pain.

Six major types of EDS exist. These types are based upon their particular symptoms and signs, with each type specifically passed on in a family. The cause of EDS is known in only three of the rare types. Ninety percent of all cases are Types I, II, and III, in which no biochemical or genetic abnormalities have yet been found. In these cases the diagnosis must be made on the basis of symptoms and family history. Fibromyalgia and chronic fatigue are common in people who have these types.

The remaining 10 percent, EDS Types IV, VI, and VII, have specific biochemical markers which can show up in laboratory tests.[7] It is unlikely that Types IV, VI, and VII will respond to guaifenesin.

Treatment is based on managing the symptoms being experienced by the individual. Surgery is sometimes needed to repair joints. Joint stability may be improved by carefully strengthening muscles.

Fibromyalgia

The word literally means pain in the muscles and fibers. But, fibromyalgia is a condition that commonly includes many more characteristic symptoms than just muscle, joint, and body pain. Despite the condition's frequency, physicians often miss the diagnosis due to the fact that there are so many other causes for most of the symptoms associated with fibromyalgia. Another confusing aspect is that the symptoms may begin following a physically traumatic event, such as an accident, surgery, or illness, leading the doctor to believe that all the symptoms are directly related to one of these events. It is now believed that these events are merely triggers that accentuate symptoms that were already building or possibly hasten symptoms that would have begun at some point in the near future anyway. Emotionally taxing events such as a death or illness of a loved one can also be triggers.

Fibromyalgia is sometimes characterized as an arthritis type condition, but this is not true because fibromyalgia does not cause inflammation and damage to the joints. Both fibromyalgia and arthritis are rheumatic conditions because they both cause joint and soft tissue pain and problems.[8]

The most common symptoms are the following:

– muscle/joint/bone pain anywhere or everywhere in the body,

including in the jaw joint, also called the temporomandibular joint, (TMJ)
- stiffness all over or in specific locations
- a general feeling of intense muscle tightness (even if the muscles are not actually tight to the examining doctor)
- an unusual sensitivity to pressure or touch in one or many places causing sufferers to avoid being touched or hugged
- headaches
- pain or sensitivity to sound, light or odors
- sleeping difficulties or unrestful sleep
- intermittent blurred vision
- itching and/or skin rashes, blemishes, pustules, and bumps
- "paper cuts" that appear on the skin and mucus membranes (mouth, nostrils, vagina and anus) for no apparent reason
- fatigue
- dizziness and balance problems at times severe
- depression, anxiety or other mood disorders
- digestive complaints, painful or frequent urination and a variety of pelvic pains
- an inability to get the arms, legs or body comfortable, especially at night
- difficulty with thought such as memory, concentration, inability to find the proper word and difficulty reading.

Additional symptoms that can involve almost any organ system in the body are also often present, and in some people may be more primary than the previously listed symptoms. All symptoms may vary greatly in intensity and duration and frequently mimic other diseases and conditions. In some cases a primary symptom may leave for no apparent reason, become intermittent, or never return. In these cases the symptom that has left is likely to be replaced, within days or months, by another symptom of similar intensity. Symptoms can be set off by an increase of physical activity, emotional stress, or a woman's menstrual cycle.

Fibromyalgia is much more common in women, approximately 80 percent of cases are female, and it tends to run in families. There are no diagnostic lab or x-ray abnormalities associated with fibromyalgia making diagnosis of fibromyalgia difficult. The symptoms ascribed to fibromyalgia cannot be due to any other medical condition, and conventional treatments and drugs provide only temporary relief. It usually takes many years for someone with fibromyalgia to be correctly diagnosed, while doctors perform tests in an attempt to determine what is wrong. Diagnosis is based upon symptoms and the presence of tender points.[9]

Because of substantial symptom overlap, many people consider chronic fatigue and fibromyalgia to be essentially the same condition. Fibromyalgia is also closely associated with other conditions, such as irritable bowel syndrome and lesser-known conditions such as neurally mediated hypotension, Raynaud's disease, and interstitial cystitis.

Irritable Bowel Syndrome (IBS)

IBS is a common "functional" disorder of the intestines. Functional means that the bowel does not work the way that it should, but that no other problem, chemical, bacterial, or structural can be found. There are no signs of disease or infection when the bowel is examined. Symptoms vary from mild to severe and are often intermittent.[10] One or a dozen different symptoms may be present including: cramping, pain, gassiness, bloating, nausea and changes in bowel habits. A common belief is that in order to have IBS, diarrhea must be a dominant symptom. This is not true. Some, but not all people with IBS have constipation, others have diarrhea, and some people experience both intermittently. Another symptom is abdominal cramps and an urge to move the bowels but without the ability to do so. A common symptom with IBS is bloating that can occur when drinking fluids, even if it is only water. This can even happen when the stomach is completely empty except for water. For most people, IBS is a chronic condition, although there will likely be times when signs and symptoms are worse and times when they improve or even disappear completely for a period of time.

Through the years, IBS has been called by many names—colitis, mucous colitis, spastic colon, spastic bowel, and functional bowel disease. Most of these terms are inaccurate. Colitis, for instance, means inflammation of the large intestine (colon). IBS, however, does not cause inflammation and should not be confused with another disorder, ulcerative colitis.

The cause of IBS is not known, and no particular test can determine the presence of irritable bowel. Diagnosis of irritable bowel depends largely upon symptoms and the lack of other conditions that can cause similar symptoms. Treatment is limited to alleviating symptoms. It is known that emotional stress does not cause a person to develop irritable bowel, but if you already have IBS, stress can trigger symptoms. IBS causes a great deal of discomfort and distress, but it is not believed to cause permanent harm to the intestines and does not lead to intestinal bleeding or to a more serious disease such as cancer. Researchers have found that the colon of a person with IBS begins to spasm after only mild stimulation, making the colon more sensitive than normal.[11]

One in five Americans has IBS, making it one of the most common disorders diagnosed by doctors. It occurs more often in women than in men, and it usually begins around age of 20.

Patients with IBS have a high frequency of non-gastrointestinal symptoms, including muscle and joint symptoms, headache, genitourinary symptoms such as urinary frequency and urgency, pain during sexual intercourse, and sleep-related disturbances.[12]

Interstitial Cystitis (IC)

IC causes discomfort or pain in the bladder and the surrounding pelvic region. Additional symptoms include a feeling of pressure, tenderness, an urgent need to urinate, a frequent need to urinate, or a combination of these symptoms. Pain resulting from sexual activity is common. These symptoms can change from time to time in an individual, and may even disappear for weeks or years before returning.[13]

Some authorities state that IC is a chronic inflammation of the bladder wall, while others do not emphasize this. Interstitial cystitis is not the same as common cystitis, which is also known as a UTI, or urinary tract infection. Urinary tract infections are caused by bacteria and in most cases respond to antibiotics. Interstitial cystitis is not believed to be caused by bacteria and does not respond to antibiotic therapy.

As little as 20 years ago, few doctors knew about interstitial cystitis, and it was considered to be a rare disease found only in postmenopausal women. Now it is known to affect any age and sex although 90 percent of cases are women. A 1997 study found that more than 700,000 people are affected in the United States. This is 50 percent more than previously thought.

Because the symptoms of IC are similar to other disorders of the bladder and pelvis, and because there is no definitive test that can identify IC, other conditions must be ruled out before a diagnosis of IC is given. It is unknown what the cause of IC is, and current treatments are aimed at relieving symptoms.

"Once patients have a diagnosis of interstitial cystitis, they are often frustrated by the lack of knowledge about IC in the medical community. Although the first IC case may have been recognized as early as the mid-1800s, it was not until 1987 that the US National Institutes of Health convened the first meeting to discuss IC. As such, patients face the unique challenge of becoming educators and advocates for the IC community, as they spread the word that IC is, indeed, a disease that is worth care and treatment."[14] IC is associated with other pelvic pain syndromes such as vulvar pain syndrome, as well as fibromyalgia, irritable bowel syndrome, and chemical sensitivities.[15]

Multiple Chemical Sensitivity (MCS)

MCS remains a medical mystery, and the medical community remains more divided over whether it really exists than it does with any of the other nonplus conditions. The Centers for Disease Control, for example, do not recognize MCS as a clinical diagnosis. This may be because symptoms and chemical exposures are often unique and are widely varied between individuals.[16]

Problems most commonly arise because of smelling perfume, paint, and dyes in clothing, or using common personal care products. Levels of exposure that are generally well tolerated by most people trigger the symptoms or signs. Exposure typically causes one or more of the following:

– immediate headache
– feeling sick or nausea
– burning sensation on the skin or face or a feverish feeling
– heart palpitations
– muscle weakness

 - mental confusion
 - difficulty breathing

These symptoms can last for minutes to days or even weeks. It occurs more commonly in women than in men. In addition, studies have shown that 40 percent of people with chronic fatigue and 16 percent of people with fibromyalgia have MCS.[17]

The diagnosis is suspected on the basis of history and physical examination, and the condition may be confirmed by removing the offending agents and rechallenging patients under properly controlled conditions. Treatment consists of avoiding offending substances.

The National Academy of Sciences estimates that 15 percent of Americans are unusually sensitive to common chemicals. Chemical sensitivity is recognized as a disability under the Americans with Disabilities Act. Multiple chemical sensitivity and Gulf War syndrome have many similarities and are possibly the same condition. However, I have no experience in treating patients with Gulf War syndrome, so I am unable to predict if guaifenesin would be helpful in these cases.

Neurally Mediated Hypotension (NMH)

The symptoms of NMH include feeling lightheaded or uncomfortable with an increase in pulse rate when sitting or standing for a prolonged time. This condition is also known as orthostatic intolerance, OI. Sometimes fainting occurs. NMH is most likely to occur in susceptible people in the following settings: after periods of quiet upright posture; after being in a warm environment; immediately after exercise; after emotionally stressful events; and after eating. Symptoms may disappear for no reason, only to return, unexplainably, days, months, or years later.

The dizziness that occurs when rising up from a lying or stooped position is commonly called "postural hypotension," and is not related to Neurally Mediated Hypotension.

NMH may be associated with decreased blood volume. Increasing fluid and salt intake often helps to reduce symptoms, but does not completely eliminate the problem. There has been information in the media that salt is unhealthful. This is not true for everyone. A strong association exists between NMH, chronic fatigue, and fibromyalgia.[18, 19]

Restless Legs Syndrome (RLS)

Restless legs syndrome was described as early as the 16th century, but was not studied until the 1940s. People with RLS complain of an irresistible urge to move their legs. This most frequently occurs during periods of inactivity and may become more severe in the evening and at night. A person with RLS can also experience pain, a vague uncomfortable feeling, or a creepy-crawly feeling that is only relieved by moving the legs. Some people explain that they move constantly in an attempt to get comfortable. The symptoms of RLS may also be present all day long, making it difficult for an individual to sit motionless. Late evening symptoms can lead to sleep onset insomnia, which tends to compound the effects of RLS. Pregnancy, uremia, and post-surgery conditions have also been known to increase the incidence of RLS.

One study found RLS to be most prevalent in middle-aged females, and its incidence increases with age. RLS tends to run in families. Though RLS is diagnosed most often in people in their middle years, many individuals with RLS can trace similar symptoms back to childhood. These symptoms may have been called growing pains.

With its classic symptoms, RLS is diagnosed by reviewing a patient's medical history. No laboratory test exists that can confirm a diagnosis of RLS. After ruling out other medical conditions as the cause of the symptoms, a healthcare provider can make the diagnosis of RLS. Restless legs syndrome is estimated to affect up to 15 percent of the population. There is no cure for this condition, and treatments are aimed at relieving or decreasing symptoms.[20]

Vulvar Pain Syndrome, Vulvodynia

Vulvodynia, also known as vulvar pain, is associated with a variety of symptoms of the external female genitalia and often occurs along with fibromyalgia, chronic fatigue, and irritable bowel. Problems can include:

- sensitivity of the skin on or around the vulva
- general discomfort from itching and dryness or a feeling of parchedness

103

- swelling and drawing sensations all over the vulvar skin or only certain parts of it, as well as in the rectal skin
- hypersensitivity along the edge of the small labia, which makes it difficult to walk
- pain or discomfort on touching or pulling pubic hair.

Some women cannot even wear underwear for these reasons. In some instances pain is primarily evoked by insertion of a tampon or by sexual intercourse. The symptoms of interstitial cystitis may also be present, as well as burning pain at the level of the pubic bone, pain in the buttocks or thighs, and pain or numbness in other areas of the body.[21]

The origin of vulvodynia is not known. Medical examinations and diagnostic workups remain unrevealing, and no specific cause of the pain can be identified. Treatment is limited to symptom relief. Preliminary findings from a Harvard Medical School study reveal that vulvodynia may affect millions of women.[22] Vulvodynia and interstitial cystitis are the most widely known conditions in a group of health problems known as chronic pelvic pain. Chronic pelvic pain can also include urethral syndrome (aching and cramping in the area above the pubic bone), coccygodynia (pain at the tip of the tailbone), low back pain or cramping, and perineal pain (pain in the pelvic floor, between the thighs). The pelvic pain syndromes share many characteristics between men and women, but with the pain centered in different locations. In men, these conditions include orchialgia (pain in the testicles), penile pain, and prostatodynia (pain in the prostate).[23]

According to Johns Hopkins School of Medicine, extreme sensitivity of the vulva was apparently a well-described subject in American and European gynecological textbooks in the 1800's. However, despite these early reports, the medical literature did not mention vulvar pain again until the early 1980s, when a new interest in this chronic pain syndrome developed. It is not clear why the chronic vulvar pain syndromes disappeared from the medical literature for almost 100 years. It is possible that the medical community denied and neglected these pain syndromes, or that chronic vulvar pain syndromes indeed were quite rare for a period of time. Further epidemiological studies are necessary to clarify these issues.

12

Additional Helpers

I have been treating the various nonplus conditions since 1982. It was not until the year 2000, however, that I saw significant and long-term improvements of all symptoms associated with the nonplus conditions as a result of using guaifenesin. But, since most symptoms improve gradually over a period of years, it is helpful to know what can be done for the symptoms that have not yet improved.

As anyone who suffers from one or more of the nonplus conditions knows, even temporary relief of just a few symptoms can be extremely difficult to find. The purpose of this chapter is to share a few of the non-guaifenesin approaches that I have learned over the past twenty-three years that may decrease or even temporarily eliminate some symptoms common with the nonplus conditions. Remember, once a person chooses to use guaifenesin, products that contain salicylates are off limits. This of course includes aspirin as well as herbal and plant-based products from aloe to valerian. If you are still unclear on the problems associated with salicylates and guaifenesin use, review Chapter 7, *The Salicylate Problem*.

Whatever successful lifestyle changes or treatments you have found useful in the past you should continue to use as long as they do not contain salicylates. Most people are already aware that some of the symptoms associated with the nonplus conditions can be decreased with the help of diet improvements, supplements, various muscle therapies, medications, exercises/stretching, and spinal, cranial, organ and extremity adjustment. In some cases, a treatment may be so effective that it resolves a particular symptom. For example, correct use of a quality magnesium supplement often eliminates constipation, even in a person who has experienced that problem for decades.

My suggestions should not be considered medical advice, and you should check with your health care provider to find which treatment or supplements are appropriate for you. The majority of the supplements or lifestyle approaches I discuss do not provide complete relief, but they can provide a safe way to decrease some symptoms. I will not be discussing prescription drug approaches. If you feel prescription drugs are necessary to control some of your more severe symptoms, discuss this with your doctor. Caution when using prescription drugs should be exercised, especially with painkillers and sleep aids, as it is common to need ever higher doses over time to maintain the same therapeutic effect. This can lead to addictions that only compound the problems already present.

The list of potentially helpful supplements is almost endless and can include almost every nutrient necessary for good health. A healthy lifestyle approach to feeling better is outlined in almost every book written on chronic fatigue, fibromyalgia, and irritable bowel, for a good reason. Sensible diet, along with consistent, appropriate exercise habits and stress management, can help anyone get the most from their body. Nevertheless, a person cannot take every supplement that has been shown to provide some health benefit. I will explain what I have learned regarding when a particular supplement is most likely to be helpful. I will also introduce several relatively unknown approaches that are frequently effective for specific symptoms.

Fatigue/Exhaustion

If you have found exercise increases fatigue, pain, and other symptoms, you are not alone. The Centers For Disease Control lists exercise induced fatigue (that is, fatigue following effort or exercise), as a defining characteristic of chronic fatigue. The notion that exercise and stretching are a bona fide treatment for chronic fatigue, fibromyalgia, or any of the nonplus conditions is something that athletes will find particularly irksome. They know that a physically active life did not prevent their health problems and that continued physical activity, although beneficial in some ways, is certainly no treatment and often only exacerbates a number of symptoms.

Many other people with a nonplus condition have a difficult time even performing routine daily activities without significant fatigue or pain, and find that most forms of exercise are all but impossible. When a doctor prescribes exercise for these people the outcome is often disastrous. After treating thousands of people, I have not seen a single person recover from one of the nonplus conditions as a result of stretching or exercising.

On the other hand, severely curtailing activity for extended periods of time will likely increase pain and disability. Exercise and stretching certainly does not treat the underlying issues, but letting your body become deconditioned because of exhaustion, pain, or any other reason will only make things worse. Some symptoms, like stiffness, depression, and difficulty sleeping, may also increase as physical activity decreases. Less exercise or no exercise also increases your risk of general health problems, such as weight gain and increased triglycerides. This puts exercise-intolerant people between a rock and a hard place.

The solution is to find exercises that only minimally increase symptoms, while providing at least some of the benefits exercise can provide. For many people this will be low intensity exercise, such as walking or riding a stationary bike, performed at a low heart rate. A good rule of thumb is to subtract your age from 180 and keep your heart rate below this number. This may help to minimize the symptoms caused by exercise while still providing the benefits. There are likely to be people who find that even this number is too high and will need to keep their heart rate even lower. Having a heart rate monitor or taking your pulse may not be necessary. Just exercise at an easy pace that is tolerable for you. What constitutes low intensity exercise varies greatly between individuals, and each person must find out what works for her.

In addition to the intensity of exercise, you have the length of time you are exercising to consider, as well as the type of exercise you choose. The usual suggestions of walking, swimming, and gentle stretches will work for a great many people. If you have been used to enjoying more intense or competitive exercise, from running to weight training, it may be emotionally difficult to scale back your activity level to what you can actually perform without causing days or weeks of pain or exhaustion.

Do not give in to the temptation of giving up completely. Be determined to do whatever little amount you can do. Even a small amount of activity will greatly reduce muscle tightness and deconditioning. If you find the exercise you prefer is no longer good for you because it causes consistent problems, find a substitute exercise that provides some of the benefit without increasing symptoms to such a degree. I have seen that using guaifenesin eventually allows most people to once again enjoy the activities they love.

When it comes to diet and nutrition, there are many products that claim to improve energy, but I have found few that actually make a difference in most people. First, let's discuss what not to do. Relying on stimulants for daily energy is not an ideal solution, and is not unlike beating an exhausted horse to increase his pace. He may go a little faster for a while, but he will collapse sooner. Prescription and non-prescription stimulants, coffee, cigarettes, and even sugary and starchy foods, can be a double-edged sword. All are addictive and can have significant side effects if used to excess, and they do not lead to long-term improvement.

I have found the most consistently effective way to increase energy is to restrict starch and sugars. Starch and sugar may lead to reactive hypoglycemia in susceptible individuals and result in a great number of symptoms, fatigue being foremost among them. I do not recommend eliminating all carbohydrates, but simply choosing healthier carbohydrates and decreasing the quantity consumed. Reactive hypoglycemia is discussed in detail in Chapter 9.

Vitamin B-12 is probably the most common deficiency I see in my practice, and will often result in poor energy and possibly several other problems. B-12 is best utilized when taken sublingually, under the tongue to dissolve slowly, because absorption through the stomach may be poor. Multiple vitamins and B-vitamins that contain B-12 may not be effective, since they are swallowed. In many cases when B-12 levels are low, energy rapidly improves with supplementation. B-12 will only help people who are low in B-12, so it is not helpful for everyone. Magnesium can result in improved energy in a small percent of people with fatigue. Many years ago, I discovered magnesium made a noticeable improvement in my energy. Because of this I started recommending magnesium to all of my patients with chronic fatigue and found that, unfortunately, it was effective for only a very few patients.

It is important to know how to take magnesium to get optimum results. Almost half of the patients I recommend to take magnesium tell me that they already are taking it or have tried it in the past. It is not until they follow these recommendations that they fully experience magnesium's positive effects. When magnesium is taken with meals, it will bind with the fat eaten during the meal. Magnesium that is bound to fat will be eliminated without being absorbed into the body. For this reason, magnesium should be taken on an empty stomach or at least when no fat has been eaten, and the daily dose can be taken all at the same time. The effective dose for most people is two to four hundred milligrams of citrate, malate, glycinate, gluconate, or aspartate. The oxide and carbonate forms of magnesium are not utilized as well, and even when taken on an empty stomach will usually require a dose about two times greater to give the same result. Magnesium will cause a loose stool if taken in excess. Taking slightly less than the amount that causes a loose stool will usually give the greatest benefit.

It is common, especially among alternative health care providers, to believe that adrenal stress or fatigue is the reason for chronic fatigue. Salivary cortisol testing and other adrenal tests may or may not disclose problems with the adrenals when chronic fatigue is present. Even when adrenal tests are positive, however, treatment with supplements geared toward resolving adrenal stress is not consistently effective in people with chronic fatigue and fibromyalgia. I spent many years trying to resolve chronic fatigue with adrenal support, and the results were disappointing in most instances. Beware that many adrenal supplements contain herbs that should not be taken if you are using guaifenesin. One of the most effective ways to treat the adrenals and increase energy is to limit sugar and starch in the diet. Lowered blood sugar brought on by reactive hypoglycemia often results in the adrenal glands being called upon to raise blood sugar via adrenaline. If the adrenals are required to frequently raise blood sugar in this way, adrenal stress and fatigue may be one result. Changing the diet to decrease sugary and starchy foods may eliminate a great deal of adrenal stress.

High potency B vitamins may significantly increase energy. Unfortunately, this effect is often short lived, and after several weeks usually wears off. Additional B vitamins taken on the days when energy is particularly bad may give more consistent results.

Sleep Difficulties

Sleep difficulties associated with chronic fatigue and fibromyalgia include: difficulty falling asleep; trouble staying asleep; restless sleep; light sleep; inability to find a comfortable position or inability to keep the body or legs in one position (restless legs); and waking up feeling exhausted even when sleep does not seem to be interrupted. Improving the quality of sleep so that you feel rested in the morning usually improves daytime energy, but not always. I have had many patients experience dramatic improvements in sleep difficulties due to using guaifenesin, but increased daytime energy may not improve at the same time.

Like so many other symptoms associated with the nonplus conditions, sleep difficulties are very difficult to treat. In some cases even the strongest prescription medications may only partially help. Because prescription sleep aids are known for their many side effects and addiction, they should be considered a last resort.

I have found that 5-HTP helps about one out of three people who try it. Although it is considered safe, it should not be taken by pregnant or lactating women without a doctor's permission. Do not use it concurrently with SSRI medications or MAO inhibitors.

B-1, also known as thiamine can be of help in some instances. In most cases sleep difficulties brought on by nonplus conditions prevent consistent, deep and restful sleep from taking place. A different type of disturbed sleep pattern may occur with B-1 need. This is characterized by several hours of normal sleep, suddenly interrupted by wakefulness and difficulty getting back to sleep. In some cases B-1 supplementation will eliminate this type of disturbed sleep. A multiple vitamin or a B-vitamin is unlikely to be of help. A B-vitamin that has more than double the amount of B-1 than B-2, or just single ingredient B-1, is more likely to be helpful with this symptom pattern. When B-1 need is the cause of this type of sleep problem, response to B-1 usually occurs within several days to one week.

Pain

I have found few supplements that can decrease the pain brought on by fibromyalgia and other nonplus conditions. One exception is pain below, beside, or between the shoulder blades. This pain is common with fibromyalgia and can feel like a rib or vertebra is out of position or that a muscle is in spasm. When this pain is due to fibromyalgia, manipulation, trigger point therapy, muscle therapies, stretching, and exercise will not provide long term relief.

A supplement called Beta TCP, made by Biotics Research Corporation, often provides more relief of this pain than other treatments including anti-inflammatory medication, muscle relaxants, and painkillers. Three per meal, or anytime the pain occurs, is often effective. Once the pain is under control, you may be able to decrease this dose or even discontinue use until the pain returns. Beta TCP contains dehydrated beet juice, vitamin C, and an amino acid. It is a potential blocker of guaifenesin, although I have had very few patients who blocked as a result of taking Beta TCP. Eating beets can also be effective, however, I have not found anyone who can manage eating beets every day.

Osteoarthritis can contribute to joint pain in people with any of the nonplus conditions. Especially if your joint pain is in the knees, hips, or shoulders you may want to try glucosamine sulfate, chondroitin sulfate, and/or MSM. It may take several months of taking these supplements before a difference is noticed.

Physical medicine such as chiropractic and physical therapy, as well as other types of body work such as massage, trigger-point therapy, and craniosacral therapy, may provide temporary and in some cases long-lasting relief in some painful areas. These procedures may also find and correct unrelated problems such as trigger points and subluxations that are contributing to nonplus conditions. People with nonplus conditions vary considerably in their tolerance to touch and pressure on the muscles, tendons, ligaments, and joints. Some people like a firmer touch, while others need a very light touch when it comes to bodywork.

It is not uncommon for individuals with the nonplus conditions to experience a mild form of Ehlers-Danlos Syndrome. This causes hypermobility in joints, a weakness or laxity in tendons and ligaments, and can contribute to joint pain, joint misalignment, joints that frequently crack and pop, and problems such as fallen arches (foot pronation). Foot pain that is the result of weakened or stretched ligaments is often relieved by a firm but slightly flexible orthotic or insole that supports the two major arches in the foot. I have found the average person does not usually need custom orthotics. Effective long lasting orthotics can cost under $100, and fit in a wide variety of shoes.

Digestive difficulties

Unlike many of the symptoms caused by the nonplus conditions, digestive difficulties are frequently helped by the correct nutritional supplement. There are many different imbalances and deficiencies that can contribute to digestive problems associated with irritable bowel. At the risk of sounding like a broken record, I have found a low carbohydrate diet to be one of the most consistently effective approaches when dealing with a wide range of digestive problems. Even if you do not have fatigue, anxiety, or some of the more common symptoms associated with reactive hypoglycemia, I recommend you consider eliminating sugar and greatly reduce starchy carbohydrate intake for two weeks if you have unresolved digestive problems. This often will result in a decrease of some and possibly many symptoms.

There are basically three types of foods that the body digests: protein, carbohydrate, and fat. If a person finds that eating one of these food groups frequently precedes the onset of symptoms, then a supplement to aid in digestion of that food group is likely to be helpful. I often ask my patients who have digestive problems what foods they avoid in order to learn what type of foods they are not digesting properly.

PROTEIN: Difficulty digesting protein is often helped by acidifying the stomach. In some cases, this can be accomplished by using vinegar at a meal or squeezing lemon or lime on food. A supplement that contains betaine hydrochloride and pepsin may be even more effective and more convenient. Although these supplements are generally considered safe and are available without a prescription, they may aggravate a sensitive stomach if not taken correctly. Check with your doctor to be sure that this supplement is for you, and how to take it.

CARBOHYDRATE: There are many digestive enzymes that aid carbohydrate digestion, and supplements designed for this purpose usually contain several. Examples are amylase, raw pancreas concentrate, and pancreatin.

FAT: Supplements that improve fat digestion are often especially helpful at relieving a variety of symptoms such as nausea, gas, diarrhea, and constipation. For people who are having difficulty digesting fat and have had their gall bladder removed, ox bile extract is often the best choice. For people with a gall bladder I recommend Beta TCP made by Biotics. This is the same supplement that I recommend for pain around the shoulder blade. When used for improved fat digestion, Beta TCP should be taken with meals.

CONSTIPATION, DIARRHEA, BLOATING, CRAMPING: I mentioned earlier that constipation can almost always be controlled with magnesium. Magnesium has several advantages over herbal laxatives, which should not be taken anyway due to the salicylate content of the herbs. Magnesium should be taken on an empty stomach when treating constipation. Start at 300 milligrams per night and gradually increase or decrease your dose by one tablet every three nights until you find the amount that allows for daily bowel movements, but without an excessively loose stool.

There are several other less common causes of constipation. Mild dehydration can cause constipation and is easily resolved by simply drinking more water and possibly consuming fewer drinks that contain diuretics, such as caffeine or alcohol. Poor fat digestion in people with or without a gall bladder can be the cause of constipation and can be greatly helped with bile salts or Beta TCP, as discussed above. A low fiber diet can contribute to constipation. Most vegetables, fruit, and whole grains are good dietary sources of fiber. If you use a fiber supplement, be sure to drink plenty of water, or constipation may actually increase. Check all ingredients in your fiber supplement to insure that it does not contain herbs or other ingredients that may contain salicylates.

Over-consumption of sugary and starchy carbohydrates may be the cause of constipation, diarrhea, and bloating in people with reactive hypoglycemia.

A deficiency of the beneficial bacteria in the colon, known as intestinal dysbiosis, may occur following the use of antibiotics. A variety of symptoms may result: constipation and/or diarrhea, gas, bloating, and cramping. Reestablishing the normal and beneficial bacteria that normally reside within the intestine may result in decreasing or eliminating these symptoms. Probiotics are foods or supplements that contain bacterial cultures that support a healthy intestinal tract. Consuming yogurt that has a seal attesting to "live and active cultures" is one way to reestablish the beneficial bacteria. Supplements are also available that contain one or several strains of beneficial bacteria. Lactobacillus acidophilus is the most well known of these bacteria. When using these supplements, best results are achieved by taking them 30 minutes before a meal.

Yeast in the gastrointestinal tract is common in my practice, and is present in people who have never had athlete's foot or a vaginal yeast infection. Yeast can cause one or all of these digestive symptoms. There are effective drugs and supplements that can eliminate yeast. One of the most effective supplements I know of for yeast in the gastrointestinal tract as well as in the sinuses, vaginal tract, and skin that is also salicylate free, is a product called SF-722, manufactured by Thorne. This nonprescription product can be taken for months if necessary, as it has few if any side effects. If yeast is causing digestive problems, the right treatment will usually cause dramatic improvement within a week or two.

Interstitial Cystitis, Vulvodynia

These problems can be debilitating physically and emotionally, because of the searing type of pain that can occur. It is known that chemicals called oxalates, found in many foods, can aggravate these symptoms, as well as caffeine and some acid-type foods. For more information on the steps that you can take to control flair-ups, go online to the Interstitial Cystitis Network and the Vulvar Pain Foundation.

Increased frequency of urination and urgency is often greatly decreased by B-1. This is another instance where a B-100 or multiple vitamin is unlikely to be helpful. What is needed is a B-vitamin that has more than double the amount of B-1 than B-2, or just single ingredient B-1. I have used this successfully on hundreds of patients.

Dizziness, Light Headedness, Postural Hypotension

These symptoms may be controlled to a certain degree by a combination of increased salt and water intake. It may be necessary for people who have been on a low-salt diet to increase salt, with the approval of their physician. Sipping from a sports type drink that contains electrolytes is often helpful. In some cases medication may be necessary to control symptoms.

13

Putting it all together

I have written this book to be different from other books on fibromyalgia or any of the nonplus conditions. Rather than offering long lists of treatment approaches, I have tried to group treatments into categories that will help you to recognize how or why a particular treatment is working. The nonplus conditions are such a complex group of health problems and symptoms that in seeking relief, most people will want to use every possible approach: lifestyle changes, symptom treatment, treating unrelated conditions that cause similar symptoms and treating cause.

With simple health problems, we use these four approaches almost instinctively and without any confusion about the purpose or limitations of each approach. When we have a more complex health issue, it is easy to get confused about what condition is causing our symptoms, which treatments will be of benefit and why a particular treatment is helping. The following example shows how each approach has its place and how, unless the cause is treated, long lasting results are difficult. I will return to the model used earlier in the book of a person getting a thorn in the foot, and how we would use the four treatment approaches for this situation.

Lifestyle adjustments: One of the first things that most people would do automatically after getting a thorn in their foot would be to make a lifestyle change by keeping weight off the foot. Limping, or using a crutch usually does this. Keeping weight off the injured area is a simple and effective way to reduce the pain. Additional lifestyle changes that optimize healing include extra rest and good nutrition. Making a lifestyle adjustment for this problem just makes good sense, but no one would suggest that it should be considered as the primary treatment for a thorn in the foot. Unfortunately, there are books, organizations, and some physicians who believe that lifestyle represents the best way to treat the nonplus conditions and imply that if you are still in pain it is because you have not modified your lifestyle enough.

Treating symptoms: If pain and swelling around the thorn became bad enough, symptom relief might be necessary with anti-inflammatory and or pain medication. Treating symptoms with medication or supplements, herbs, etc., is often necessary and can be a great help in almost every health problem. There is no advantage, however, to using this approach to the exclusion of the others. When it comes to treating the nonplus conditions, you will likely find doctors who will emphasize this treatment approach to the exclusion of the other three.

Treating unrelated conditions that cause similar symptoms: If it was not obvious that a thorn was in the foot or if the thorn was not visible it would be reasonable to consider other possible reasons for continued pain. There are other conditions that can cause a sharp stabbing pain in the sole of the foot. Three possibilities are athletes foot, fallen arches (foot pronation) which can cause a sharp pain in the arch or heel and dropped metatarsals that occur in the fore foot that can cause a sharp pain in the ball of the foot. Treating one or all of these conditions, if they were present would help to reduce some of the pain in the foot but would do nothing to relieve pain that was caused by the thorn.

Treating Cause: Unless the cause of the problem is addressed by pulling out the thorn, the other treatment approaches become an ongoing necessity. Once the thorn is pulled out, most of these approaches are no longer necessary or are only needed for a short time. To a certain extent, the same is true for using guaifenesin to treat the nonplus conditions. As guaifenesin allows recovery to occur, symptoms decrease and symptom management with drugs, supplements, and reduced activity becomes less necessary.

Of course, diagnosing, treating and managing any one of the nonplus conditions is much more complex than a thorn in the foot. Pulling out a thorn is a simple and fast process while taking guaifenesin and recovering from the nonplus conditions is a long term, possibly lifelong process. In spite of this, taking guaifenesin is similar to removing the thorn in the sense that both treat the cause and greatly reduce the need for the other treatments.

If for some reason you decide not to use guaifenesin or if you are one of the approximately 20 percent of the people who do not respond to guaifenesin, then an understanding of the four treatment approaches will still be very important for you. In addition, knowledge of the relationships between the nonplus conditions should be helpful in understanding why you are experiencing so many different types of symptoms.

There is a saying that I hear from many of my more senior patients, "Getting old isn't for sissies." When I hear that I always reply with, "Yes, but it is better than the alternative." Likewise, I know for a fact that the nonplus conditions are not for sissies. Fortunately, much can be done to reduce symptoms and even reverse the conditions themselves.

I wish everyone with one or more of the nonplus conditions much success in using each treatment approach and taking back control of your health and your life.

Bibliography

Introduction
1. Goldenberg DL. Fibromyalgia and related syndromes. In: Hochberg MC, Silman AJ, Smolen JS, Weinblatt ME, Weisman MH, eds. *Practical Rheumatology*. 3rd ed. Philadelphia, PA: Mosby; 2004: 255.
2. Clauw DJ. Fibromyalgia. In: Ruddy S, Harris ED, Sledge CB, eds. *Kelley's Textbook of Rheumatology*. 6th ed. Philadelphia, PA: W.B. Saunders, 2001: 421.
3. Jason LA, Richman JA, Friedberg F, et al. Politics, Science, and the Emergence of a New Disease: The Case of Chronic Fatigue Syndrome. *Am Psychologist*. 1997; 52:973-983.
4. James LF. *The Rise and Fall of Modern Medicine*. New York, NY: Carol & Graf Publishers; 2000: 16-25.

1: Understanding fibromyalgia, chronic fatigue, irritable bowel and the other nonplus conditions
1. *Webster's New Collegiate Dictionary*. Springfield, MA: G & C Merriam Co; 1977.
2. U. S. Food and Drug Administration Center for Drug Evaluation and Research. Letter to the author: CDER/ DrugInfo – RC; 8-27-04.
3. Clauw DJ. Fibromyalgia. In: Ruddy S, Harris ED, Sledge CB, eds. *Kelley's Textbook of Rheumatology*. 6th ed. Philadelphia, PA: W.B. Saunders, 2001: 418.
4. Goldenberg DL. Fibromyalgia and related syndromes. In: Hochberg MC, Silman AJ, Smolen JS, Weinblatt ME, Weisman MH, eds. *Practical Rheumatology*. 3rd ed. Philadelphia, PA: Mosby; 2004: 255.
5. James LF. *The Rise and Fall of Modern Medicine*. New York, NY: Carol & Graf Publishers; 2000: 147-156.

6. Richman JA, Jason LA, Taylor RR, Jahn SC. Feminist Perspectives on the Social Construction of Illness States. *Health Care For Women International*. 2000; 20: 173-185.
7. Clauw DJ. Fibromyalgia. In: Ruddy S, Harris ED, Sledge CB, eds. *Kelley's Textbook of Rheumatology*. 6th ed. Philadelphia, PA: W.B. Saunders, 2001: 421-422.

2: Treating the Nonplus Conditions

1. *Drug Facts and Comparisons*. St. Louis, MO: Wolters Kluwer Health, Inc; 2006.
2. Munger R. Guaiacum, the Holy Wood from the New World. *Journal Of The History of Medicine and Allied Sciences*. 1949; 4: 205-206.
3. Jason LA, Richman JA, Rademaker AW, et al. A community-based study of chronic fatigue syndrome. *Archives of Internal Medicine*. 1999; 159: 2129-2137.
4. U. S. Food and Drug Administration News. FDA Proposes Steps to Assure the Safety and Efficacy of Certain Currently Unapproved Medicines. 10-17-2003; Available at: www.fda.gov/bbs/topics/NEWS/2003/NEW00962.html Accessed April 15, 2006.

3: Guaifenesin Rediscovered

1. Clauw DJ. Fibromyalgia. In: Ruddy S, Harris ED, Sledge CB, eds. *Kelley's Textbook of Rheumatology*. 6th ed. Philadelphia, PA: W.B. Saunders; 2001: 417.
2. Hazelman B. Soft-tissue rheumatism. In: Maddison PJ, Isenberg DA, Woo P, Glass DN, eds. Oxford Textbook Of Rheumatology. 2nd ed. Oxford: Oxford University Press; 1998: 1496.
3. Copeman WSC. Historical. In: Copeman WSC, ed. *Textbook Of The Rheumatic Diseases*. 3rd ed. Edinburgh: E. & S. Livingstone LTD; 1964: 3.

4. Campbell SM, Wernick R. Update in Rheumatology. *Annals of Internal Medicine*. 1999; 130: 135-142.

5. Rubin E, Farber JL. *Pathology*. 3rd ed. Philadelphia, PA: Lippincott; 1999: 1405.

6. Theodosakis J. *The Arthritis Cure*. New York, NY: St. Martin's Press; 1997.

7. Copeman WSC. Historical. In: Copeman WSC, ed. *Textbook Of The Rheumatic Diseases*. 3rd ed. Edinburgh: E. & S. Livingstone LTD; 1964: 3.

8. Munger R. Guaiacum, the Holy Wood from the New World. *Journal Of The History of Medicine and Allied Sciences*. 1949; 4: 205-206.

9. Wright V, Moll JMH. *Seronegative Polyarthritis*. Amsterdam: North-Holland Publishing Company; 1976: 1.

10. Goldenberg DL. Fibromyalgia and related syndromes. In: Hochberg MC, Silman AJ, Smolen JS, Weinblatt ME, Weisman MH, eds. *Practical Rheumatology*. 3rd ed. Philadelphia, PA: Mosby; 2004: 255.

11. Mathew B, ed. *CITES* (Convention on International Trade in Endangered Species of Wild Fauna and Flora) *Guide to Plants in Trade*. CITES: Department of Environment; 1994.

12. World Conservation Monitoring Centre. *Guaiacum sanctum*. Tree Conservation Database; 1998.

13. Munger R. Guaiacum, the Holy Wood from the New World. *Journal Of The History of Medicine and Allied Sciences*. 1949; 4: 196-229.

14. St. Amand P. *What Your Doctor May Not Tell You About Fibromyalgia*. New York, NY: Warner Books; 1999.

15. Aspirin Foundation of America. History. Available at: www.aspirin.org/history.html Accessed April 14, 2006.

16. *Drug Facts and Comparisons*. St. Louis, MO: Wolters Kluwer Health, Inc; 2006.

4: Nonplus Conditions: Different Symptoms One Cause
1. Goldenberg DL. Fibromyalgia and related syndromes. In: Hochberg MC, Silman AJ, Smolen JS, Weinblatt ME, Weisman MH, eds. *Practical Rheumatology.* 3rd ed. Philadelphia, PA: Mosby; 2004: 258.
2. Veale D, Kavanagh G, Fielding JF, Fitzgerald O. Primary fibromyalgia and the irritable bowel syndrome: different expressions of a common pathogenetic process. *Br J Rheumatol.* 1991; Jun; 30(3):220-2.
3. Davis C. Arthritis Foundation, 2004. What's In A Name: Fibro vs. CFS. Available at: http://www.arthritis.org/resources/news/news_fibro_cfs.asp Accessed April 14, 2006.
4. Clarke DA. Ehlers-Danlos National Foundation. Learning To Manage Fibromyalgia Syndrome. Available at: http://www.ednf.org/abouteds/content/view/156/49/ Accessed April 14, 2006.
5. Clauw DJ. Fibromyalgia. In: Ruddy S, Harris ED, Sledge CB, eds. *Kelley's Textbook of Rheumatology.* 6th ed. Philadelphia, PA: W.B. Saunders; 2001: 418, 422-424.
6. Ehlers-Danlos Support Group. What Are The Types of EDS? Available at: http://www.ednf.org/abouteds/content/view/13/31/ Accessed August 14, 2006.
7. Clauw DJ. Fibromyalgia. In: Ruddy S, Harris ED, Sledge CB, eds. *Kelley's Textbook of Rheumatology.* 6th ed. Philadelphia, PA: W.B. Saunders; 2001: 417.
8. St. Amand P. *What Your Doctor May Not Tell You About Fibromyalgia.* New York, NY: Warner Books; 1999.
9. Copeman WSC. Historical. In: Copeman WSC, ed. *Textbook Of The Rheumatic Diseases.* 3rd ed. Edinburgh: E. & S. Livingstone LTD; 1964: 3.

5: Phosphate Retention Theory

1. St. Amand P. *What Your Doctor May Not Tell You About Fibromyalgia*. New York, NY: Warner Books; 1999.
2. Copeman WSC. Historical. In: Copeman WSC, ed. *Textbook Of The Rheumatic Diseases*. 3rd ed. Edinburgh: E. & S. Livingstone LTD; 1964: 2,3,4.

7: The Salicylate Problem or step one: avoiding salicylates

1. Delaney TP, Uknes S, Vernooij B, et al. A Central Role of Salicylic Acid in Plant Disease Resistance. *Science*. 1994; 266:1247-1250.
2. St. Amand P. *What Your Doctor May Not Tell You About Fibromyalgia*. New York, NY: Warner Books; 1999.
3. Heinicke RM, Van der Wal M, Yokoyama MM. Effect of bromelain (Ananase) on human platelet aggregation. *Experientia*. 1972; 28:844-845.
4. Morita AH, Uchida DA, Taussig SJ. Chromato graphic fractionation and characterization of the active platelet aggregation inhibitory factor from bromelain. *Arch Inter Phar Ther*. 1979; 239: 340-350.
5. Livio M, Bertoni MP, De Gaetano G, et al. Effect of bromelain on fibrinogen level, prothrombin complex factors and platelet aggregation in the rat – A preliminary report. *Drugs Under Experimental and Clinical Research*. 1978; 4: 49-53.
6. Maurer HR. Bromelain: biochemistry, pharmacology and medical use. *Cellular and Molecular Life Sciences*. 2001; 58(9): 1234-45.

9: Reactive Hypoglycemia
1. National Institute of Diabetes and Digestive and Kidney Diseases, (n.d.). Hypoglycemia. Available at: http:// diabetes.niddk.nih.gov/dm/pubs/hypoglycemia/ Accessed April 14, 2005.
2. Merck Manual, 2004. Hypoglycemia. Available at: http:// www.merck.com/mrkshared/mmanual/section2/chapter13/ 13e.jsp Accessed April 14, 2006.
3. Genter PM, Ipp E. Diabetes Care. *American Diabetes Association.* 1994; 17(6): 595-598.

10: Frequently Asked Questions
1. James LF. *The Rise and Fall of Modern Medicine.* New York, NY: Carol & Graf Publishers; 2000: 26-51.
2. Harvie D. *Limeys.* Gloucestershire: Sutton Publishing; 2002.
3. *Drug Facts and Comparisons.* St. Louis, MO: Wolters Kluwer Health, Inc; 2006.
4. U. S. Food and Drug Administration News. FDA Proposes Steps to Assure the Safety and Efficacy of Certain Currently Unapproved Medicines. 10-17-2003; Available at: www.fda.gov/bbs/topics/NEWS/2003/NEW00962.html Accessed April 15, 2006.
5. U. S. Food and Drug Administration Center for Drug Evaluation and Research. Letter to the author: CDER/ DrugInfo – RC; 8-27-04.
6. Dieppe D, Schumacher RH, Wollheim Jr. FA. *Classic Papers in Rheumatology.* London: Martin Dunitz; 2002: 227.
7. St. Amand P. *What Your Doctor May Not Tell You About Fibromyalgia.* New York, NY: Warner Books; 1999:157-160.
8. Ibid.

9. Copeman WSC. Historical. In: Copeman WSC, ed. *Textbook Of The Rheumatic Diseases*. 3rd ed. Edinburgh: E. & S. Livingstone LTD; 1964: 2,3,4.
10. Goldenberg DL. Fibromyalgia and related syndromes. In: Hochberg MC, Silman AJ, Smolen JS, Weinblatt ME, Weisman MH, eds. *Practical Rheumatology*. 3rd ed. Philadelphia, PA: Mosby; 2004: 259.

11: Defining the Nonplus Conditions
1. Chronic Fatigue and Immune Dysfunction Syndrome Association of America, 2004, "Symptoms," http://www.cfids.org/about-cfids/symptoms.asp Accessed April 13, 2006.
2. Ibid.
3. Centers For Disease Control and Prevention. Chronic Fatigue Syndrome. http://www.cdc.gov/ncidod/diseases/cfs/treat.htm Accessed April 13, 2006.
4. Jason LA, Richman JA, Friedberg F. Wagner L, Taylor R, Jordan KM. Politics, Science, and the Emergence of a New Disease. *American Psychologist*. 1997; 52: 973-983.
5. University of Maryland Medicine, 2001, "What Causes Chronic Fatigue Syndrome?" http://www.umm.edu/patiented/articles/what_causes_chronic_fatigue_syndrome_000007_3.htm Accessed 2004 Oct. 3.
6. University of Washington, Seattle. Ehlers-Danlos Syndrome-Symptoms. http://www.orthop.washington.edu/uw/tabID_3376/ItemID_32/mid_10313/PageID_4/Articles/Default.aspx Accessed April 13, 2006.
7. Ehlers-Danlos National Foundation. How is EDS Diagnosed? http://www.ednf.org/abouteds/content/view/29/32/ Accessed April 13, 2006.

8. National Institute of Arthritis and Musculoskeletal and Skin Diseass. What Is Fibromyalgia? http://www.niams.nih.gov/ hi/topics/fibromyalgia/fibrofs.htm#fib_a Accessed April 13, 2006.

9. Ibid.

10. Mayo Clinic. Irritable bowel syndrome. http:// www.mayoclinic.com/invoke.cfm?objectid=F32C84B7-11F3-4E9D-80A5AD5354F27F4E&dsection=2 Accessed April 13, 2006.

11. National Digestive Diseases Information Clearing House. Irritable Bowel Syndrome. http://digestive.niddk.nih.gov/ ddiseases/pubs/ibs/ Accessed April 13, 2006.

12. Whorwell PJ, McCallum M, Creed FH, Roberts CT, et al. Non-colonic features of irritable bowel syndrome. *Gut.* 1986; 27:37-4.

13. National Institute of Diabetes and Digestive and Kidney Diseases. Interstitial Cystitis. http://kidney.niddk.nih.gov/ kudiseases/pubs/interstitialcystitis/index.htm Accessed April 13, 2006.

14. Interstitial Cystitis Network. Interstitial Cystitis, The History of IC. http://www.ic-network.com/handbook/ basics.html Accessed April 13, 2006.

15. Alagiri M, Chottiner S, Ratner V, Slade D, Hanno PM. Interstitial cystitis: unexplained associations with other chronic disease and pain syndromes. *Urology.* 1997; 49(5A Suppl): 52-57.

16. National Institute of Environmental Health Sciences. Allergies: Multiple Chemical Sensitivities. http:// www.niehs.nih.gov/external/faq/allergy.htm Accessed April 13, 2006.

17. The Merck Manual. Multiple Chemical Sensitivity Syndrome. http://www.merck.com/mmhe/sec25/ch306/ ch306d.html Accessed April 13, 2006.

18. National Fibromyalgia Research Association. Neurally Mediated Hypotension in Fibromyalgia Patients. http://www.nfra.net/NewRowe1.htm Accessed April 13, 2006.
19. Chronic Fatigue and Immune Dysfunction Syndrome Association of America. Medical Journal Articles. http://www.cfids.org/youth/articles/medical/nmh.asp Accessed April 13, 2006.
20. University of Pittsburgh Medical Center. Restless Leg Syndrome. http://restlesslegsyndrome.upmc.com/Treatment.htm Accessed April 13, 2006.
21. The Vulvar Pain Foundation. A Word About Vulvar Pain. http://www.vulvarpainfoundation.org/vpfabout.htm Accessed April 13, 2006.
22. Harvard Medical School, 2003 April. Chronic Vulvar Pain May Be a Highly Prevalent Disorder. http://www.hms.harvard.edu/news/pressreleases/bwh/0403chronic_vulvar_pain.html Accessed April 13, 2006.
23. Johns Hopkins Medicine. Chronic Pain Syndromes in Women. http://www.neuro.jhmi.edu/PelvicPain/home.html Accessed April 13, 2006.

Index

Symbols

5-HTP 110

A

acetylsalicylic acid 33, 53–58. *See also* aspirin
acupuncture 17
adjustments 40, 106
adrenal stress and fatigue 109, 110
adrenaline 68, 110
allergic reaction 60
aloe 56, 84, 105
American College of Rheumatology xviii, 39
Americans with Disabilities Act 102
amylase 113
antibiotics 15, 19, 100, 114
aquarium phosphate testing kit 81
arthritis 30, 83, 97. *See also* osteoarthritis, rheumatism
Aspercreme 55
Aspergum 57
aspirin vii, 33, 53, 56, 57, 83. *See also* salicylates
Atkins Diet 72

B

B vitamins 110
B-1 vitamin 111, 115
B-100 vitamin 115
B-12 vitamin 20, 108, 109
B-2 vitamin 111, 115
Balfour, William 39
Ben Gay 57
Beta TCP 111, 113, 114
betaine hydrochloride 113
biliary stasis 20
Biotics Research Corporation 111
blood sugar 67–73, 110. *See also* glucose, reactive hypoglycemia
bromelain 57

Index

O

o-carboxyphenol 55
octyl-salicylate 55
orchialgia 104
osteoarthritis 30, 31, 33, 83, 111
ox bile extract 113

P

pancreatin 113
pelvic pain syndromes 94, 101, 104
pepsin 113
peptic ulcers 9
perineal pain 104
periodic limb movement disorder 36, 94
phosphate retention theory 43, 45, 46, 48, 55, 63, 80, 86
phosphates 43, 44, 46, 48, 49, 50, 86
phosphorus 43
physical therapy xvii, 3, 112
plasma half-life 77
Plavix 57
postural hypotension 36, 102, 115
Practical Rheumatology 5, 121, 123
Primary Raynaud's 94
probiotic supplement 19, 114
prostatodynia 104
protein 71, 72, 73, 96, 113
psychological counseling 17

Q

quinine 30, 31, 93

R

Raynaud's disease 99
reactive hypoglycemia vii, 13, 22, 33, 51, 52, 67–73, 84, 108, 110, 112, 114
restless legs syndrome v, 9, 12, 38, 93, 103
rheumatism 24, 29, 30, 31, 32, 33, 39, 45, 83
rheumatoid arthritis 30, 31, 33, 83
rheumatology xviii, 5, 15, 24, 30, 39
RLS. *See* restless legs syndrome

S

sacroiliac ligament strain 18
salicylate-free products vii, 55, 57, 58
salicylates vii, 25, 27, 33, 34, 44, 45, 46, 51, 52, 53–58, 61, 62, 65, 82–88, 105, 114
salivary cortisol testing 109
scurvy 14, 76, 77
sensitive bowel. *See* irritable bowel syndrome
SF-722 114
South Beach Diet 72
SSRI medications 110
St. Amand, Paul 32, 39, 43, 54, 80
sulfur 30, 31, 33
symptoms. *See* see many specific references

T

The Rise and Fall of Modern Medicine 76
The Textbook of the Rheumatic Diseases 30
thiamine 111
thoracic subluxation 20
thyroid 8, 12, 90, 91
Ticlid 57
trigger points 13, 20, 43, 91, 112
triglycerides 107

U

ulcers 9, 15, 89
uremia 103
urethral syndrome 104
uric acid 33, 34, 45, 46
uricosuric medications 34
urinary tract infection 100
US National Institutes of Health 101

V

vitamin C 76, 77, 111
vitamins, multiple 109
Vulvar Pain Foundation 115
vulvar pain syndrome 36, 101, 103
vulvodynia v, 2, 12, 36, 103, 104, 115

Y